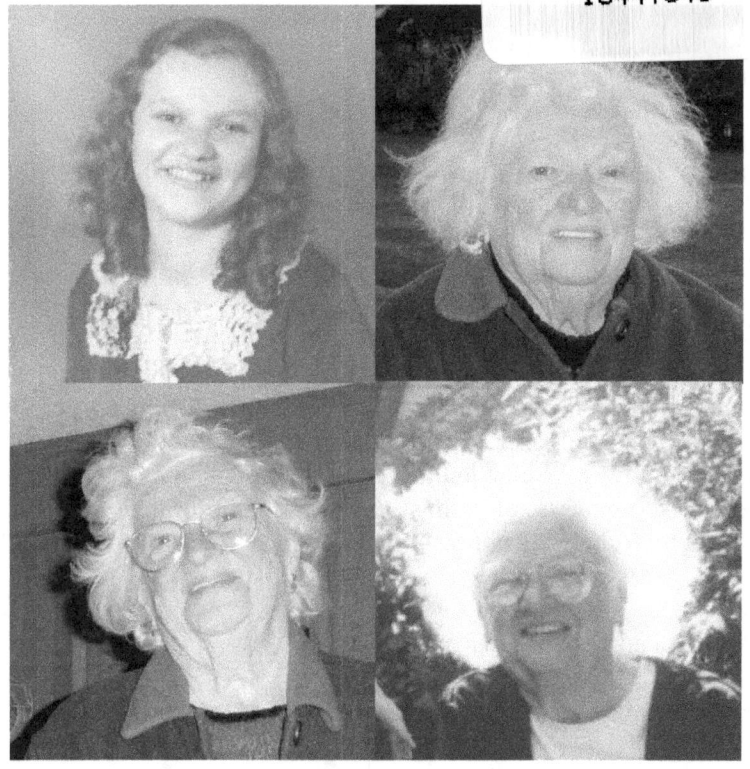

Alzheimer's--What My Mother's Caregiving Taught Me

"Essential Knowledge for Effective Caregiving"

by Robert J. Bublitz

Title Page

Self-Published through CreateSpace, a DBA of On-Demand Publishing LLC, Part of the Amazon group of companies.

Book design and photos by Robert Joseph Bublitz

Library of Congress Cataloging-in-Publication Data

Bublitz, Robert Joseph, 1942-

Includes biographical references.

Paperback ISBN-13: 978-1479116164 and ISBN-10: 1479116165
eBook (Kindle) ISBN:

Book Industry Standards and Communications (BISAC) Subject Code:
Health & Fitness / Diseases / Alzheimer's & Dementia

Search Keywords:
1. Alzheimer 2. Dementia 3. Caregiving 4. Aging 5. Elderly Disease

Book's Internet URL: http://www.alzheimerwhatmomscaretaughtme.com

Printed in the United States of America

Preface

The primary goal of this book is to help Caregivers; Health Care, Legal, Insurance and Financial Professionals; and Social Workers understand and deal with Alzheimer's disease by describing Olive Mae Bublitz's journey. The secondary goal is to educate the public about the current health care crisis. Everyone should be aware of Alzheimer's since most people will care for an aging parent or grandparent or deal with the disease themselves once they reach age eighty. The book accomplishes these goals by: (1) Providing a history of Alzheimer's; (2) Elaborating on the behaviors to expect during each of the seven stages; (3) Describing Olive's history with Alzheimer's; (4) Making recommendations for caregivers and (5) Providing extensive resources in the Appendix.

This book is organized into nine sections: an introduction, seven chapters that parallel the seven stages of Alzheimer's disease and a conclusion. Each of the inside seven chapters describes: (1) Common behaviors for each stage; (2) Descriptions of Olive's experience and (3) Recommendations. Additionally, extensive appendixes for reference include: (1) Essential Caregiver Information; (2) Example Legal Documents: Will, Trust, General Power of Attorney, Health Care Directive, Do Not Resuscitate Order (DNRO) and Final Arrangements; (3) Diagnosing Guidelines; (4) List of National Alzheimer Disease Research Centers; (5) Olive's Clinical Diagnosis (6) Hospice Patient Re-Qualification Worksheets; (7) Olive's Certificate of Death and Autopsy Results; (8) Collage of Olive's Life; (9) Olive's Obituary & Eulogy; (10) Condolence e-Mail from a Friend; (11) Useful References and (12) Author Profile. Appendix A includes: (1) Declining Memory Assessment; (2) Driver Reality Check; (3) Key Documents Summary; (4) Alzheimer's Patient Care Checklist; (5) Alzheimer Support Team Contact List; (6) Working Agenda for Caregiving Meetings; (7) Net Worth Calculation; (8) Monthly Income and Expense Budget; (9) Board & Care and Nursing Home Evaluation.

Alzheimer's--What My Mother's Caregiving Taught Me

People reading this book will gain a better understanding of the disease and information on how to effectively care for a loved one with Alzheimer's. I believe knowledge is power. Your experience may differ in terms of the duration of the stages, difficulties, and behaviors you experience. My intent is pure and simple education, to reach out and share our experience to help others deal with this dreadful terminal disease.

I almost did not document this care because it is so painful. However, I feel it is important to write about Alzheimer's because it is such a devastating disease. I think it is more painful than death. At least death is final. Alzheimer's Disease is insidiously long, unpredictable and is challenging financially, emotionally and spiritually. During this long period of the disease, I watched the light at the center of my existence slowly dim and vanish. Watching mother experience difficulty with household chores and repeating questions was painful and often confusing. During November 2001, Olive was involved in an auto accident. Following an examination at The Mayo Clinic, everything became clear. Olive was diagnosed with Alzheimer's disease.

In the early stage, there were little miracles when portholes opened and we were able to have normal, rational conversations. Then Olive would go away. In March of 2005, I returned to sell Olive's home to help pay for accumulating medical and care expenses. This family home was a special place for over sixty years. It was just the way Olive had left it in February 2002 with its 1960's décor. Olive's furniture was all in the same place. Her beautiful oil paintings hung proudly from the walls. The drapes she had so carefully sewn graced the windows. Olive was committed to preserving her memory for our lives.

During the final phase of Olive's Alzheimer's, she developed paranoia, would hallucinate and experience motor, vision and eating complications and pain. However, there were times when mother would show glimpses of her old self. One day in June 2007 when Mother heard my voice, she woke right up from a nap. After a brief hug and a kiss, I sat down next to mother and we shared a period of silence. Then I took some index cards from my shirt pocket and reading from my notes on the cards, reviewed the wonderful things Olive had done during her life and told her how blessed she was with many caring friends. I had prepared these notes on index cards earlier in the month because I knew this would make Mother feel good. She would be happy as she always was in the past. She listened intently as she looked out in the distance. After I finished reading the note cards, Mother turned, looked directly at me, smiled and blew me two quick kisses. Afterwards, I pushed her around the back yard in her wheel chair. As we stopped in front of each blooming rose bush, I pulled the flowers over to her so she could see them better and enjoy their fragrance. Late that afternoon I took the picture of Mother, which is displayed in Figure 38: Olive and son, Bob, Leisure Living, November 19, 2005 on page 136. Two months later mother passed away.

During the last two years of mother's life, she stopped walking, had to be fed and used non-verbal communication because she could not talk. Eventually, with many difficulties, she died at age 87.

May this written and photo description of Olive's journey, along with the extensive appendix, improve your understanding and allow you to provide quality care. Your own research, organizational preparedness and support network are also vitally important. Together they will provide you with the power to withstand the tremendous stress of this disease.

Other than the birth and parenting of my two daughters, I consider this book to be the most significant work of my life. I hope that it will prove indispensable in caring for people facing Alzheimer's.

This book is dedicated to a very special person in my life, my mother, Olive Mae Bublitz (August 5, 1920 to August 15, 2007).

Bob Bublitz, Author
Bob.Bublitz@gmail.com
4400 Sevenoaks Court
Westlake Village, CA 91361

Book Statistics:
Pages/File Size: 319/276 Mb
Word Count: 63063
Lines/Paragraphs: 9491/3711

Acknowledgements

First, I want to thank The Mayo Clinic for their diagnosis of Olive's Alzheimer's conditions. Additionally, I want to especially thank Dr. David S. Knopman, M.D. Neurology for the generous time he took to examine and consult with mother and me. This diagnosis allowed us to make long-term plans for Olive's affairs and care. Additionally, I would like to thank the following people:

- Cousins Don & June Voss for looking after Olives affairs, inviting her to their home for holidays and for helping me move furniture. Don & June went above the call of duty and cared for Olive like their own mother. Additionally, I want to thank Don and June for describing situations with heir parents and allowing me to use them in this book.
- Howard and Betty Dailey for their support and for describing situations with their father, my Uncle Ray, and allowing me to document them in this book.
- Larry and Lana Bublitz and Dan and Karen Bublitz, for their support and for describing situations with their father and my first cousin Elmer and allowing me to document them in this book.
- Nellie Kemp and Darlene Schaefer of Elkhorn, WI for their weekly visits while mother was still living in her home.
- Dr. Edward B. Portnoy, M.D. and Dr. Razmig Krumian, D.O. of Westlake Village, CA who routinely provided check-ups and prescriptions.
- Maureen Simon and Senior Concerns staff for the extensive program they provided Olive.
- Sue Lindeman, Facilitator of the Alzheimer's Support Group in Thousand Oaks and all its members for sharing their insights in providing care.
- Ross and Pam Hashemi, Owners of Leisure Living and their caring, thoughtful, attentive staff.
- Ana Barajas and Claribel Montenegro, Caregivers.
- Bonnie Olson, President of Buena Vista Hospice and her staff.

Acknowledgements

- Neighbor Rhonda & Jeff Zimmerman who looked out for Olive.
- Dick Howrath, Attorney for meeting with the city and disposing of the Bublitz Case Company Factory.
- Roger & Alice Eisele for visiting mother when I was out of state, listening to plans for this book, suggestions, proofreading and encouragement.
- Grant Davis, who I have worked with over the years, for his frequent telephone calls, help on many issues including this book, advice, concern and keeping my spirits positive and my thoughts creative during my recovery from cancer while caregiving for Olive.
- Friends Jim Lindauer and Ken Vensel for their friendship.
- Ken Bayus, Carlsbad, CA for his numerous phone calls, visits, providing mother with frequent bouquets of beautiful roses and always willing to lend a hand where he was able. Ken's thoughtful condolence eMail is included beginning on page 300.
- My daughters Aubrey and Shelby for their weekly phone calls and visits.
- Neighbor, John Madison for advice he gained from also caring for his mother with Alzheimer Disease, taking me grocery shopping while I recovered from cancer surgery and being a thoughtful neighbor.
- Neighbors, Bob & Caroline Raser. Bob for his frequent afternoon visits and discussions while I was recovering from cancer surgery. Bob was mourning the loss of his mother to breast cancer. Bob produced a DVD of an Alzheimer's Consultation Session. Caroline for the quality of her questions during a recording of the Alzheimer's Consulting Session concerning care for her mother who is in the early stage of dementia.
- Lifelong friends Dr. Leon Helmbrecht, Urologist for his medical advice during my bout with cancer. Pastor Sam Platts for his spiritual offering.
- Carol Suminski for her disciplined quality proofreading and her valuable suggestions of the manuscript on five complete readings of the book.
- Last and most important, my life long friend, Kirt Fiegel and his wife Dixie for their advice and support. Without Kirt and Dixie, I would not have made it through this experience alive.

Table of Contents

Table of Contents

Table of Contents

Table of Figures

Note to the Reader

Robert J. Bublitz, author of this book, describes his caregiving experience with his mother Olive. Mr. Bublitz is not a licensed health care, legal, insurance, financial or social work professional. Although this information should be useful in many Alzheimer care situations, the author cannot tell you whether or not the information is right for you because every individual circumstance is different. If you want advice geared to your specific situation, consult an expert. General information is not a substitute for personalized advice from a knowledgeable health care, legal, insurance, financial or social work professional licensed to practice in your state.

The author and publisher cannot accept responsibility for any loss, injury or damage caused as a result of the contents of this book; nor for any proceedings instigated against any person or body that may result from this book's contents.

Introduction

Background

This book emerged from the sixty-eight month experience being the primary caregiver for my mother, Olive, who suffered from Alzheimer's disease. Each chapter covers an overview of common behaviors in each of the seven stages of the disease, Olive's experience, caregiving and recommendations. The appendix includes extensive references. In addition to textual descriptions, you can also view the decline from the photos.

It is my intent that this book be straightforward, easy to understand and able to be read in a single day.

Alzheimer's Disease

Alzheimer's is a neurodegenerative disease typically found in people over age 65. Approximately 24 million people worldwide have dementia, formerly known as senility. Dementia diseases include Alzheimer's, Vascular Dementia, Parkinson, Creutzfeldt-Jacob, Huntington's or Pick's disease and Lewy Bodies. Sixty percent of dementia disease may be classified as Alzheimer disease.[1]

Alzheimer's disease (AD) is caused by plaques containing misfolded proteins called beta amyloid that formed in the brain many years before the

---

[1] National Institute of Health.

clinical signs of Alzheimer's are observed. Together, these plaques and neurofibrillary tangles form the pathological hallmarks of the disease.[2] In Alzheimer's disease, these unusual proteins build up in and around neurons in the neocortex and hippocampus, parts of the brain that control memory. When these neurons die, people lose their capacity to remember and their ability to do everyday tasks. Physical damage to the brain and other parts of the central nervous system can also kill or disable neurons.[3]

Vascular Dementia is the second most common type of dementia. Alzheimer's disease and vascular dementia often occur together. In fact, some scientists believe that it is more common for these two disorders to occur together than apart. Vascular dementia is an umbrella term that describes impairments in cognitive function caused by problems in the blood vessels that feed the brain. In some cases, a blood vessel may be completely blocked, causing a stroke. Some strokes result in dementia while others do not. It depends on the severity of the stroke and the portion of the brain that is affected. Vascular dementia also can occur when blood vessels in the brain narrow, reducing the amount of blood flow to those sections of the brain.[4]

Currently about 5 percent of men and women age 65 have AD, and nearly half of those age 80 and older may have the disease.[5] The prevalence of vascular dementia ranges from 1 percent to 4 percent in people over the age of 65. The risk increases dramatically with age. Vascular Dementia, a type of dementia caused by brain damage from cerebrovascular or cardiovascular problems, usually results in strokes. According to the National Institute of

[2] Mayo Clinic on Alzheimer's Disease, Ronald Peterson, M.D., Ph.D., Editor in Chief and head of the Neurology Department, Mayo Clinic, Rochester, Minnesota, Published 2002.
[3] National Institute of Neurological Disorders and Stroke, Institute's Brain Resources and Information Network (BRAIN), P.O. Box 5801, Bethesda, MD 20824, (800) 352-9424
[4] Mayo Foundation for Medical Education and Research (MFMER), May 1, 2007.
[5] National Institute of Health Publication Number 06-3431, dated July 2006.

Neurological Disorders and Stroke, vascular dementia accounts for up to 20 percent of all dementias.[6]

Alzheimer's Care Cost

The cost of care for an Alzheimer's patient in the early mild or moderate stage of Alzheimer's, who is cared for by the family and lives in the community, is estimated at $80,852 per. year. Similarly, as the disease progresses to the severe stage, the annual cost climbs to $109,995. Alternatively, if a person is institutionalized, the annual cost is $107,593. Total cost of care for an Alzheimer patient living in the community for three years and institutionalized for three years is approximately $572,541. Similarly, living in the community for three years in the early stages, one year in the severe stage and three years in an institution is $756,182. Family provided costs are based on replacement cost if a nursing assistant, housekeeper, bookkeeper and handyman provided the services. An alternative approach is to use the lost opportunity cost for the estimate. In this case you use the cost associated with the work you gave up to care for the loved one. A list of the caregiving tasks that the family provides is on page 27.

---

[6] National Institute of Neurological Disorders and Stroke, National Institutes of Health, Bethesda, MD 20892.

2008 Type of Living	Stage of Alzheimer's	Annual per Person Family Provided Care Cost	Annual per Person Medical & Social Care Cost	Total Annual Cost per Person	6-Year Total Cost per Person	8-Year Total Cost per Person
Community	Mild to Moderate	$62,916	$17,936	$80,852	$242,556	$323,408
	Severe	71,686	38,309	109,995	329,985	109,995
Institution		10,918	96,675	107,593		322,779
					$572,541[7]	$756,182

Figure 1: Cost of Alzheimer's Care [8]

Alzheimer's - High Probability when Born After 1950

Figure 2 on page 20 should signal an alarm to anyone born after 1950, of the crisis taking place in the United States with Alzheimer disease during a person's elder years. The average life span for anyone born after 1950 is well into his or her eighties. Nearly half these people will, according to present day statistics, face Alzheimer's. This is why it is so urgent to support the Alzheimer Association to find a treatment for this dreadful disease. Insuring that a certificate of death accurately reflects the cause of death when

---

[7] Note: Six year total cost includes three year in a mild stage living in the community and three years in an institution. Eight year total cost includes four years living in community during the mild to moderate phase, one year during the severe stage and three years living in an institution.

[8] Source: Alzheimer's Disease Facts and Figures in California, Alzheimer Association, February 2009 and Rice, DR, Fox, P J, Max, W, Webber, P, Lindeman, D, Hauck, W, & Segura, E (1993). The Economic Burden of Alzheimer's Disease Care, Health Affairs, Volume 12, Issue 2, 164-176.

a person dies from Alzheimer disease is very important. The certificate of death is used to determine how research funding is allocated.

AGE	65	70	75	80
Probability of Alzheimer	5%	10%	20%	40%

Figure 2: Probability of Alzheimer's Between Age 65 & 80

During the course of the Alzheimer's disease, a person progresses through the following seven stages:[9]

- Stage 1: No impairment (normal function).
- Stage 2: Very mild cognitive decline may be normal age-related changes or the earliest signs of Alzheimer's disease.
- Stage 3: Mild cognitive decline.
- Stage 4: Moderate cognitive decline, may be mild or early-stage Alzheimer's disease.
- Stage 5: Moderately severe cognitive decline may be moderate or mid-stage Alzheimer's disease.
- Stage 6: Severe cognitive decline may be moderately severe or mid-stage Alzheimer's disease.
- Stage 7: Very severe cognitive decline may be severe or late-stage Alzheimer's disease.

The person afflicted with Alzheimer's usually notices symptoms of the disease beginning in stages two or three, and develops backup systems to compensate for the problems associated with the disease. Close friends or relatives and loved ones usually recognize the memory decline of Alzheimer's when it is in Stage four or five. The disease may last as long as

---

[9] Source: The Alzheimer Association Internet Site, September 2008, Alzheimer's Association National Office 225 N. Michigan Ave., Fl. 17, Chicago, IL 60601 or http://www.alz.org.

twenty years. Typically, it takes six to eight years to go from diagnosis in stage five to the end of a person's life in stage seven.

Alzheimer's Disease is Currently Terminal!

The Time Lines of the key events during Olives Alzheimer's are described in Figure 3 and Figure 4 on page 36 and 37. These time line diagrams describe Olive's decline with Alzheimer's disease relative to the various phases of the disease published and described by the Alzheimer Association.

My experience began November 2001, when mother was involved in an auto accident and her local doctor suggested mental testing because she did not seem her normal self. January 2002, I flew from Los Angeles to Chicago's Midway Airport and on to mother's home in Elkhorn, Wisconsin. After spending a few days with mother in early 2002, we drove to The Mayo Clinic in Rochester, Minnesota for a scheduled neurology department assessment to see if there was brain injury resulting from the auto accident.

Like the handling of mother's cardiac problems ten years earlier, we decided to go to The Mayo Clinic in Rochester, Minnesota because of the success Olive experienced with the analysis and treatment of her cardiac condition. Additionally, according to the Annual U.S. News and World Report Survey of Best Hospitals in the America, The Mayo Clinic is ranked number one or two in nearly every medical category. In Neurology & Neurosurgery The Mayo Clinic ranks #1 and in Heart & Heart Surgery #2.[10]

---

[10] U.S. News and World Report, July 2008 issue. Posted on the Internet July 10, 2008, at http://health.usnews.com/sections/health/best-hospitals. U.S. News analyzed data on 5,453 medical centers to produce this year's 16 specialty rankings. Only 170 hospitals were ranked in one or more specialties and, of those, just 19 were of Honor Roll caliber. To be in this elite group, which rewards breadth of excellence, a hospital had to achieve high scores in six or more specialties. The order is based on points—a hospital earned 2 points for ranking at or close to the top in a specialty, 1 point if ranked slightly lower. The ranking are: #1 Johns Hopkins Hospital, Baltimore; 30 points in 15 specialties; #2 Mayo Clinic, Rochester, MN, 28 points in 15 specialties; #3 Ronald Reagan UCLA Medical Center, Los Angeles, 25 points in

Additionally, we chooses The Mayo Clinic for the same following reasons that a half a million people from around the world choose the clinic:[11]

- Top doctors
- Pioneer in new treatments
- Reputation for solving difficult medical issues
- Many viewpoints
- Single Location, Quality, Efficient & Superior Medical Care

As usual, the diagnosis was thorough, professional, timely and thoroughly documented for the patient to understand. We then sat down with a neurologist after the testing. After general introductions and conversation, he turned to mother and said, "Olive, there is good news and bad news." Olive said, "I'd like to hear the good news first." The neurologist then proceeded to tell her, "Olive, the good news is, there is no brain injury from the accident." She then stated, "Well, then what is the bad news?" The neurologist stated, "The bad news is, after reviewing your brain MRI, you have a fairly advanced case of Alzheimer's disease and will no longer be able to live alone." The impact of the diagnosis was beyond Olive's comprehension.

Mother was always one of the primary and most important supporters in my life. When it came to her cardiac problems in the early nineties, I dropped everything, consulted with a lifelong friend, Leon, who became a urologist, and then sought a diagnosis and found an effective treatment at The Mayo Clinic. In seeking a solution for her memory problems my approach was similar. Go to one of the best medical facilities in the world, get a diagnosis, find an effective treatment, and continue with the enjoyment of life. This time it was different. Alzheimer's disease turned out to be much more challenging since effective treatment is not available for this terminal disease. Also, unbeknown to me, the disease is at a national crisis level

---

14 specialties; 4 Cleveland Clinic, 25 points in 13 specialties; and #5 Massachusetts General Hospital, Boston, 24 points in 12 specialties.

[11] See Appendix E: Why Patients Choose The Mayo Clinic for more information.

because of the number of people being diagnosed. Furthermore, the cost of caring for a loved one with the disease can range from five hundred thousand dollars to over a million dollars. In many cases Alzheimer's care will completely consume every family asset, energy and patience. Also, dealing with the associated stress of the disease is very difficult for the immediate family. Sometimes the stress level is beyond what a family is capable of enduring. Currently, half the caregivers develop significant health conditions or die before the loved one because of the extreme stress. The emotional, financial, and spiritual demands are beyond what most people experience with anything else in their entire lifetime. In mother's case, I was determined to help her beat this health setback just as we did with the heart problems. Unfortunately, it was much different. After the diagnosis of Alzheimer's disease, I tried to read every available book, article, pamphlet or handout available in print form or on the Internet. At the outset of the experience, I had only a vague idea of the meaning of Alzheimer's and how to care for someone suffering from this disease. Due to my extensive reading, conversations with other caregivers, involvement with caregivers at support groups and knowledge gained from medical professionals and other research, I decided to share the knowledge I gained. I hope this information helps others understand the disease and effectively care for their loved ones. May this book help every reader go forward and be better prepared to handle the exhausting demands of this disease with better understanding, known alternatives and the ability to get more out of life.

Alzheimer's Risk Factors

According to the National Institute of Health, "Scientists do not yet fully understand what causes Alzheimer's disease. There probably is not one single cause, but several factors that affect each person differently. The risk factors for Alzheimer's disease include the following:

Age

Age is the most important known risk factor for Alzheimer's disease. The number of people with the disease doubles every five years beyond age

65."[12] The older people get, the more likely they will be diagnosed with Alzheimer's disease.

Genetics (heredity)

Scientist have identified the gene, apolipoprotein E-e4 (APOE-e4) which causes early-onset Alzheimer's disease, a rare form of Alzheimer's disease that occurs between the ages of 30 and 60 which is inherited.[13]

The majority of AD cases are late-onset, usually developing after age 65. Late-onset AD has no known cause and shows no obvious inheritance pattern. However, in some families, clusters of cases are seen. Although a specific gene has not been identified as the cause of late-onset AD, genetic factors do appear to play a role in the development of this form of AD. Only one risk factor gene has been identified so far.

Researchers have identified an increased risk of developing late-onset AD related to the apolipoprotein E gene found on chromosome 19. This gene codes for a protein that helps carry cholesterol in the bloodstream. The APOE gene comes in several different forms. Three occur most frequently: APOE e2, APOE e3, and APOE e4.

To help identify the genes that play a role in the development of Alzheimer's disease, the National Institute on Aging has funded the National Cell Repository for Alzheimer disease. This national resource is a place where clinical information and genetic material (DNA) can be stored from individuals with Alzheimer's disease as well as from individuals without any

---

[12] First published: 19 March 2002, Last reviewed: 12 March 2007, NIH Senior Health, National Institute on Aging, U.S. National Library of Medicine, National Institutes of Health, U.S. Department of Health & Human Services.

[13] Alzheimer's Disease Genetics Fact Sheet, Last reviewed: 24 July 2008, NIH Senior Health, National Institute on Aging, U.S. National Library of Medicine, National Institutes of Health, U.S. Department of Health & Human Services. Additional information is available from the National Human Genome Research Institute (NHGRI), part of the NIH. Visit the NHGRI website at www.genome.gov. The National Library of Medicine's National Center for Biotechnology Information also maintains genetic information at: www.ncbi.nlm.nih.gov/disease

symptoms of memory loss or dementia.

Diabetes

"It has been known for some time that type 2 (adult) diabetes is a risk factor for Alzheimer's disease. It was generally assumed that this was because the blood vessel and heart disorders associated with diabetes are also risk factors for Alzheimer's disease."[14]

Head Injury

Blows to the brain, or the damage caused by a stroke, can kill neurons outright or slowly starve them of the oxygen and nutrients they need to survive.[15] Brain injuries, especially repeated concussions, and damage caused by stroke are risk factors for the later development of Alzheimer's disease.

Heart-Head Relationship

"Scientists are finding more clues that some of the risk factors for heart disease, strokes and "mini strokes," like high blood pressure, high cholesterol and low levels of the vitamin folate may also increase the risk of Alzheimer's."[16]

Alzheimer's Prevention

- Protect Your Head from Potential Accidental Blows
- Eat Nutritious Meals
- Maintain Your Weight at the Target Level for Age and Height
- Avoid Tobacco Products

---

[14] Risk Factors for Alzheimer's Disease: A Prospective Analysis from the Canadian Study of Health and Aging, American Journal of Epidemiology 2002; Vol. 156, No. 5, 445-453.
[15] National Institute of Neurological Disorders and Stroke, Institute's Brain Resources and Information Network (BRAIN), P.O. Box 5801, Bethesda, MD 20824, (800) 352-9424
[16] First published: 19 March 2002, Last reviewed: 12 March 2007, NIH Senior Health, National Institute on Aging, U.S. National Library of Medicine, National Institutes of Health, U.S. Department of Health & Human Services.

- Do Not Drink Alcohol in Excess
- Stay Socially Connected
- Exercise Both Your Body and Mind
- Reduce Exposure to Pesticides, Herbicides, Fertilizer, Food Preservatives and Air Born Pollutants

CAREGIVING

The dictionary defines the word caregiver[17] as:

care·giv·er [káir gìvvər]

(plural care·giv·ers)

noun

1. Individual who looks after somebody: the individual who has the principal responsibility for caring for a child or dependent adult, especially in the home. Also called caretaker

U.K. term carer

2. Somebody assisting in management of illness: a medical or other professional who assists in the management of an illness or disability

Since Alzheimer's has no cure and it gradually renders patients incapable of tending to their own needs, caregiving essentially is the treatment. It must be carefully managed over the course of the disease.

During the early and moderate stages, modifications to the patient's living environment and lifestyle can increase patient safety. Taking the car keys away from a loved is one of the most traumatic events for the person with Alzheimer's because it limits their freedom and independence. However, it is necessary to protect them and others from injury.

As the disease progresses, different medical issues can appear, such as oral and dental disease, pressure ulcers, malnutrition, hygiene problems, respiratory, skin, nail or eye infections. Careful management of the patient can help prevent many of these medical issues, while professional treatment is needed when they do arise. When swallowing difficulties begin, the use of

---

[17] Microsoft Encarta Reference Library 2005.

a feeding tube is debated from both an evidence-based and an ethical point of view. The use of physical restraints is rarely indicated in any stage of the disease, although there are situations when they are necessary to prevent harm to the patient or their caregivers. During the final stages of the disease, treatment is centered on relieving discomfort until death.

Caregiving Tasks

The assistance provided by a loved one for the person afflicted with Alzheimer's varies depending on the needs of the individual and the stage of the disease. Caregiving tasks may include the following:

- Round-the-clock supervision
- Supervision of others who provide care
- Lifting, bathing, dressing, grooming, mobility, feeding, toilet and incontinence care
- Helping the person take medication correctly
- Housekeeping, shopping for groceries, preparing meals and providing transportation
- Making arrangements for medical care, paid in-home care, board and care or skilled nursing home and hospice care
- Supervising the person to avoid unsafe activities such as wandering and getting lost, driving, etc.
- Managing finances and legal affairs
- Outdoor and indoor maintenance
- Social activities, listening, talking, and providing emotional support
- Managing behavioral symptoms

Coping with Caregiving

Caregiving is a difficult job and many caregivers show symptoms of psychological stress and decline in physical and mental health, especially when caregiving continues over two years time, which is usually the case with Alzheimer's. Below are some of the difficulties caregivers experience.[18]

Emotional Stresses
- Concern over the care recipient's health and safety
- Changes in household roles such as household financial management, meal preparation, and keeping in touch with friends and relatives
- Change in identity due to the addition of a caregiving role and reductions in employment due to caregiving
- Loss of friends and supports due to increased time in caregiving
- Feelings of depression
- Feelings of anger and resentment about the change in the loved one and the caregiving role
- Feelings of guilt about wanting personal time or about feeling angry when the loved one needs care

Physical Stresses
- Loss of sleep and fatigue from being constantly attentive and alert
- More health problems due to the caregivers aging and the demands of caregiving

Financial Problems
- Worries about inadequate insurance coverage and about paying for nursing home care
- Leaving the labor force to care for elderly relatives, lost wages, lost opportunity to earn a higher income and lower retirement benefits
- Spouse's distress over the future impact of their illness on their mate

Stress, Stress Reduction, Problem Solving, Attitude & Grieving

Stress
Hans Selye,[19] endocrinologist at the University of Wisconsin was the first

---

[18] Alzheimer's Caregiver Support Online (Alzonline) is a telehealth project sponsored by the State of Florida Department of Elder Affairs and the University of Florida (UF) Center for Telehealth, http://www.alzonline.phhp.ufl.edu

person to use the term "stress." Selye found there are three stages to stress: (1) Alarm, (2) Resistance and (3) Exhaustion. The first stage, when the threat or stress is identified or realized, the body's stress response is a state of alarm. During this stage, adrenaline will be produced in order to bring about the fight-or-flight response. There is also some activation of the hypothalamic-pituitary-adrenal or HPA axis, producing cortisol. The HPA axis, a major part of the neuroendocrine system controls reactions to stress and regulates many body processes, including digestion, the immune system, mood, emotions, sexuality, and energy storage and expenditure. Resistance is the second stage. If the stressor persists, it becomes necessary to attempt some means of coping with the stress. Although the body begins to try to adapt to the strains or demands of the environment, the body cannot keep this up indefinitely, so its resources are gradually depleted. Exhaustion is the third and final stage. At this point, all of the body's resources are eventually depleted and the body is unable to maintain normal function. At this point the initial autonomic nervous system symptoms may reappear (sweating, raised heart rate, increased blood pressure, etc.). If stage three is extended, which it usually is with Alzheimer's caregiving, long term damage may result as the capacity of glands, especially the adrenal gland, and the immune system are exhausted and function is impaired.

The result can manifest in illnesses such as ulcers, depression, diabetes, trouble with the digestive system, cardiovascular problems, and mental illnesses. This is the primary reason why so many caregivers end up with substantial health problems or death as a result of Alzheimer's caregiving.

Stress Reducing Strategies
The following three strategies are described here for reducing stress while

---

[19] Several books by Hans Selye are available from libraries and on Amazon. The results of his research findings are described at the Wikipedia Internet site at, http://en.wikipedia.org/wiki/Stress_(biological).

---

caregiving for a person with Alzheimer's:[20]

- Change lifestyle
- Get an early diagnosis and develop a manageable caregiving plan for your loved one with AD
- Seek relief through relaxation

Change our lifestyle

- Get enough sleep
- Eat nutritiously
- Exercise regularly[21]
- Plan your day
- Simplify your schedule
- Get organized
- Take occasional breaks
- Change the pace
- Be positive
- Stay connected with family and friends
- Be patient

Relief Through Relaxation Techniques

- Meditation[22]
- Breathing
- Guided Imagery

Manage your caregiving problems

This will be described in more detail under the next heading.

---

[20] Mayo Clinic on Chronic Pain (Control Your Pain Instead of Allowing It To Control You) (Paperback), Mayo Clinic (1999), 178 pages.

[21] See Walking: The Ultimate Exercise for Optimum Health in Appendix M: Useful Alzheimer's References on page 307.

[22] See Appendix N: Useful Alzheimer's References for Dr. Andrew Weil's Mind-Body Tool Kit, which describes proven techniques for breathwork, meditation, guided imagery & sound therapy on page 308.

Introduction

Problem Solving Process

The problem solving process is an important concept in Alzheimer's caregiving and consists of the following steps:[23]

1.   Identify the Problem
2.   Identify and Create Alternatives and Options
3.   Evaluate Alternatives
4.   Anticipate Negative Consequences & Chaotic Times
5.   Overcome Obstacles to Carry out a Solution
6.   Choose A Solution & Develop a Caregiving Plan
7.   Monitor the Solution
8.   Evaluate the Success of the Plan

The following is an elaboration on each of the above steps:

1.   Identify the Problem

The first step is knowing the real problem or issue which is half the battle. A diagnosis at an AD Research Center is essential.

2.   Identify and Create Alternatives and Options

Once a diagnosis at an AD Research Center is reached, brainstorming by the family should generate options or alternatives surrounding the identified problem.

3.   Evaluate Alternatives

Ask what your family thinks of each of the options. Each family member should give his/her opinion of the idea. Eliminate the alternatives that the family is unwilling to try. The goal is to find an option that each family member will agree to consider. Next, decide whether or not the family can afford that option.

---

[23] Families First-Keys to Successful Family Functioning: Problem Solving, Publication Number 350-091, June 1999, Authors: Rick Peterson, Extension Specialist and Assistant Professor, Department of Human Development, and Stephen Green, Graduate Student, Department of Human Development, Virginia Tech and Epstein, N. B. Bishop, D., Ryan, C., Miller, & Keitner, G., (1993) The McMaster Model View of Healthy Family Functioning. In Froma Walsh (Ed.), Normal Family Processes (pp. 138-160). The Guilford Press: New York/London.

4. Anticipate Negative Consequences & Chaotic Times

5. Overcome Obstacles to Carrying out a Solution

6. Choose A Solution & Develop a Caregiving Plan

    Once you have evaluated all the alternatives, decide as a family which idea or ideas you are willing to pursue. This is known as the Caregiving Plan which includes each action item, person responsible, timing and cost. Putting the plan in writing enables everyone to better understand the plan and their part in the caregiving and resolving problems or issues.

7. Monitor the Solution

    Critical to the problem-solving process is monitoring the effectiveness of the Caregiving Plan which also allows your family to keep track of their progress.

8. Evaluate the Success of the Plan

    This stage involves reviewing what happened in order to learn from the situation. The review helps the family to make adjustments to the plan and to evaluate what worked and what didn't.

Positive Attitude

Prior to this change, we were comfortable because our situation was familiar. We resist change due to fear of the unknown. As we move toward new roles and routines, we may experience feelings of fear, anger, sadness or resistance as well as relief, hope or excitement. It may feel confusing and chaotic, but it can also be a time of creativity and challenge. What we do with these feelings makes the difference. When we're able to find something positive or see possibilities, we'll have energy and motivation to take the next step.

Thoughts + Feelings = Reaction

We choose how to respond to our thoughts and feelings. This determines our behavioral or emotional reaction to change, whether positive or negative.

We cannot change the past or how others act, but we can change our attitude. William James, the father of modern psychology, said, "The most important discovery of our time is that we can alter our lives by altering our attitudes." If we learn to manage our attitudes, we won't feel paralyzed and the benefits will follow. These benefits include:

- Being a positive role-model for your children and others
- An increase in self esteem along with an increase in productivity
- An increase in energy
- A better lifestyle
- Spending final quality time with the family member
- Time to reevaluate your goals
- Meeting new people and learning new things
- Imagining the additional possibilities

Grieving

Grieving, along with the problem solving process and your attitude as a caregiver, is very important in understanding the Alzheimer's journey. Grieving is something you as a caregiver and the person diagnosed with Alzheimer's will experience off and on during the various stages of Alzheimer's. The Kübler-Ross model best describes the stages of Grieving:[24] The following is an adaptation of this model for Alzheimer's Caregiving purposes:

- Confirmation.
  Example: Following a diagnosis, "At least we now know what we face and we develop a plan for care."

- Denial.
  Example - "I feel fine. This can't be happening, not to me!"

---

[24] Adapted from Kubler-Ross, E (1973) On Death and Dying, Routledge, ISBN 0415040159. Kubler-Ross, E (2005) On Grief and Grieving: Finding the Meaning of Grief Through the Five Stages of Loss, Simon & Schuster Ltd, ISBN 0743263448. Stages one and seven have been added to this model by the author. Also, see Kübler-Ross model at the Wikipedia Internet site.

- Anger.

  Example - "Why me? It's not fair!" Or "NO! NO! How can this happen!"

- Bargaining.

  Example - "Just let me live to see my children graduate." Or "I'll do anything, can't you stretch it out? A few more years."

- Depression.

  Example - "I'm so sad, why bother with anything?" Or "I'm going to die . . . What's the point?"

- Acceptance.

  Example - "It's going to be OK."

- Hope.

  Example: Hope for the future is always important for the afflicted and especially the caregiver.

Caregiving Rewards

- Accepting Responsibility and Obligation
- Expression of Love
- Increased Sense of Confidence and Self-worth When Tasks are Mastered
- Sense of Accomplishment
- Development of a Closer Relationship

Caregivers usually feel a responsibility and obligation to help an older family member and find many joys and rewards from caregiving.[25] Spouses often feel that caregiving is part of the responsibility they accepted when they were married; it is an expression of love that is treasured by the care recipient. Husbands in particular may feel a need to express gratitude to their wives for their support and devotion to the home and family in the earlier years of the marriage. Caregivers who master new tasks feel an increased

---

[25] Alzheimer's Caregiver Support Online (Alzonline) is a telehealth project sponsored by the State of Florida Department of Elder Affairs and the University of Florida (UF) Center for Telehealth, http://alzonline.phhp.ufl.edu

sense of confidence and self-worth. Adult children who are caregivers usually help their parents willingly and feel satisfaction and a sense of accomplishment. Children may develop a closer relationship with their parents while sharing time and providing care; they may even be relieved to resolve old conflicts. Parents may express more appreciation of their adult children than they have in the past. Children may strengthen their relationships with brothers or sisters who are helping.

Conclusion - Most Love Ones Accept Caregiving

Most caregivers don't want a way out of caregiving. They see this as a responsibility, a time to repay their spouse, parents or friends for the support and care provided in earlier years. However, caregiving places numerous emotional, physical, and financial demands on caregivers. In addition, employed caregivers often feel that they are holding two full-time jobs, their eight-to-five employment and their caregiving. To protect their personal health and economic resources, caregivers must find ways to reduce stress to cope with caregiving so that they will be able to meet their caregiving, work, and family demands and enjoy the many aspects of their lives.

Time Line of Olive's Alzheimer's

	STAGE 1	STAGE 2	STAGE 3
	Normal Age Related Memory Changes		
Cognitive Decline	No Impairment	Very Mild	Mild
Key Activities	• Owned Own Home in Rural Small Town & Lakeside Cottage • Husband dies Nov 1973 • 1987, 10-year Relationship ends	• Late 1980's Stopped Painting • 1990s Commun-ication Begins to Lose Effectiveness • Asset Assessment • Review Legal Docs • Inventory Personal Property	• Hospitalized Multiple Times for Rapid Arrhythmia • Last CA Visit 12/95 • Passed Mini Mental Exam • Financial Plan • Credit Report
Olive's Age	<67	68-73	74-77
Duration	Prior to 1987	1988-1993	1994-1997
Living Type	Own Home	Own Home	Own Home

Figure 3: Time Line of Olive's Life before Alzheimer's, 1 of 2

	STAGE 4	STAGE 5	STAGE 6	STAGE 7
	Alzheimer's Related Memory Changes			
Cognitive Decline	Moderate Early-Stage Alzheimer's	Moderately Severe **Cognitive**	Severe **Functional**	Very Severe **Behavioral**
Key Activities	• Concussion from Fall, Double Vision for 24-months • Auto Accident 11/2001	Diagnosis Jan 2002[26] • Full Neuro-Psy. testing • Brain MRI • Attend Sr. Concerns • Physical 6-months • Sold Lake Property	• Physical Qtly. • Son's HELOC • Sold City Property • Son's Cancer Diag. 12/05 • Cancer Srgy. 2/06 • Dr. Orders Hospice 5/06	• Hospice May 2006 • Applied for Medicaid, SS, VA • Cardiac & Hypertensio n Meds Stopped April 06 • Morphine for Osteoporosis Pain May 06
Olive's Age	79-81	81-83	84-85	86 to 87 & 10-days
Duration	1998-2001	2002-09/2005	10-11/2005	05/06-Died 8/15/2007[27]
Living Type	Own Home	Son's Home Board & Care[28]	Board & Care	Board & Care

Figure 4: Time Line of Olive's Life with Alzheimer's, 2 of 2

---

[26] See Diagnosing Alzheimer's Disease on page 239. On the average, people with Alzheimer's live for eight to ten years after diagnosis. Some live as long as twenty years. Olive lived sixty-eight months after diagnosis or five years and eight months to age 87.

[27] U.S. Average Life Span for women born during the 1920 is 78 and men 77.

[28] November 10, 2004, Olive moved to a private board and care home.

Stage 1

Stage 1: No Impairment/Normal Function

Typical at Stage 1: Unimpaired individuals who experience no memory problems and none are evident to a health care professional during a medical interview.[29]

Olive was born to Joseph Skotzke and Evelyn Albright Skotzke in Burlington, Wisconsin. Olive's father worked as a manager for the Burlington Woolen Mills. Before Olive entered grade school, the family moved to Milwaukee, Wisconsin and eventually resided on Oakland Avenue in Shorewood, a Milwaukee suburb. Joseph owned a tailor shop one block from the family home. Olive grew up in Shorewood and graduated from Shorewood University High School

---

[29] All "typical at stage" comments are from The Alzheimer Association Internet Site, September 2007 and are in bold italics unless otherwise noted at the beginning of the next six chapters. Alzheimer's Association National Office 225 N. Michigan Ave., Fl. 17, Chicago, IL 60601 or http://www.alz.org. Also, the author recommends each reader obtain a free copy of, Caring for a Person with Alzheimer's Disease, Your Easy-to-Use Guide from the National Institute on Aging, NIH Publication Number: 09-6173, May 2009. A free copy of the book maybe obtained by contacting the Alzheimer's Disease Education and Referal Center (ADEAR) at 1-800-438-4380 or by the internet: http://www.nia.nih.gov/Alzheimers.

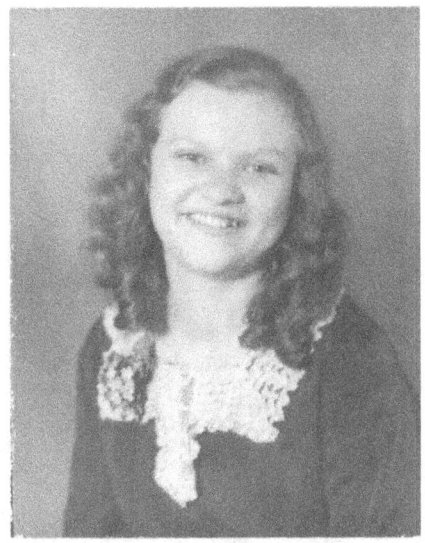

Figure 5: Olive at Age 16

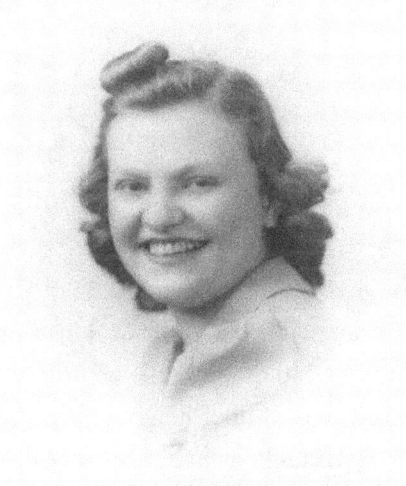

Figure 6: Olive's Shorewood University High School Graduation Photo, Age 19

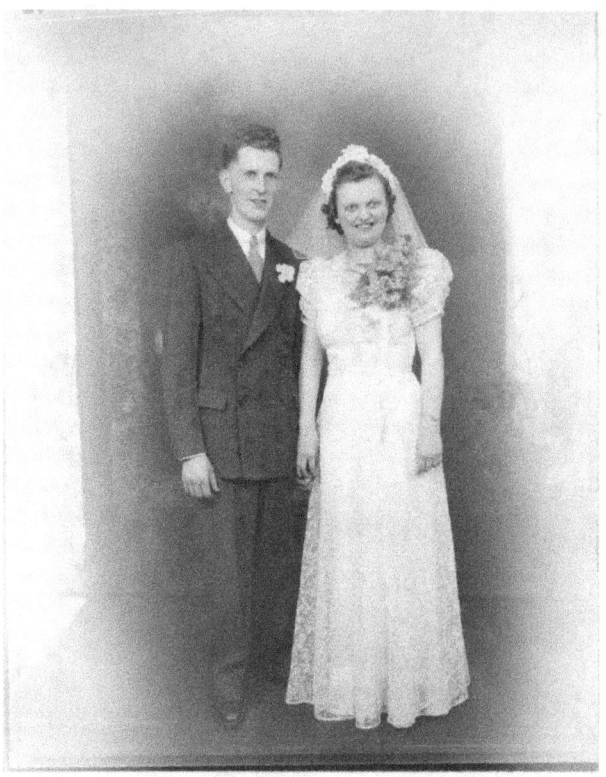

Figure 7: Olive & Her Husband, Bob on Their Wedding Day, April 19, 1941

In the early forties Olive met and married Robert Earnest Bublitz who was involved with the manufacturing of musical instrument cases with his brother Bill. Olive and Bob built their home on property next to the factory in Elkhorn, Wisconsin. The next-door neighbor was Brother Bill. Uncle Gus and Grandmother Tina lived in the next house east of Brother Bill. During her teens, Olive was healthy except for problems with her left ear, which caused her family to seek frequent medical attention. On one occasion, a mastoid[30] was removed from her left ear, which resulted in hearing loss as she grew older. Later in her teens, Olive came down with Rheumatic Fever.[31] The effects from the Rheumatic Fever developed into life long heart problems. These problems became more severe at age fifty-four, following her husband's sudden fatal heart attack.

Olive's husband Bob entered the military service shortly after they were married during World War II. A year after Olive and Bob were married, Olive gave birth to their son, Bob. The pregnancy was difficult and Olive eventually had to deliver her son via a cesarean section. The operation left Olive unable to bear additional children. During World II, Olive and I traveled back and forth between her mother's home in Milwaukee and her mother-in-law's home fifty miles away in Elkhorn, Wisconsin. After Bob returned from serving in World War II, he resumed work with his brother Bill, manufacturing musical instrument cases. Immediately Olive and Bob started to build a house. During this time, Olive's father suffered a massive heart attack and died. He was only 60 years old. I can remember up through third grade coming home and mother would be crying due to the loss of her father and concern for her mother who was still suffering from the effects of being hit by a streetcar. Olive was in her early teens when the accident happened and her mother needed medical attention for the injuries until she was in her 60's. She did finally fully recover and lived to be 93. As time

---

[30] Up until the 1950s, mastoiditis was quite common and a major cause of death in American children. Treatment of mastoid inflammations typically required either a simple mastoidectomy, in which part or all of the mastoid process was removed, or a radical mastoidectomy, in which the eardrum and most of the structures of the middle ear were removed. Today antibiotics are widely used to treat infections of the middle ear, and serious mastoid infections are far less frequent. As a result, a mastoidectomy is seldom performed. Microsoft ® Encarta ® Reference Library 2005.

[31] Rheumatic fever is an inflammatory disease that may develop after an infection with Streptococcus bacteria (such as strep throat or scarlet fever). The disease can affect the heart, joints, skin, and brain. MedlinePlus, A service of the U.S. National Library of Medicine, 8600 Rockville Pike, Bethesda, MD 20894, 20894, National Institutes of Health, Department of Health & Human Services.

passed, Olive and her husband, Bob completed building their home, the business grew and life was quite idyllic from the mid forties through the sixties.

During this time, Olive and Bob worked from Monday through Friday in the musical instrument manufacturing business next to their home. Olive handled complex tasks with efficiency and was busy between the business and household chores. Each year, a summer company picnic was held in our backyard for approximately thirty to forty employees. At Christmas, there was a luncheon in the factory. Olive prepared all the food for each event. Employees looked forward throughout year for these two events. Friday night's, Olive and Bob usually enjoyed a fish fry at a local restaurant with either friends or relatives. Saturday night, during the entire marriage, Olive and Bob went dancing. Around the house, Olive would frequently hum or sing songs. When she and Bob would take breaks, they would occasionally dance briefly or simply hug. There was a lot of camaraderie between Olive and her husband Bob; in work, handling family household chores, relaxation and recreation. My parents shared a deep love for one another. Olive enjoyed cooking[32] and was always looking for flavorful tasty recipes as well as keeping their house immaculate. In her spare time Olive enjoyed being with friends, playing cards, practicing or giving brief concerts on either the piano or organ, sewing, rose mauling, oil painting, gardening and genealogy.

During the summer of 1972, my parents and Uncle Gus drove from Wisconsin to Oregon to visit my wife Nina and I for a couple of weeks, stopping and visiting Yosemite on the way. Figure 8 on page 43 is a picture of son Bob, brother-in-law Gus, husband Bob, daughter-in-law Nina and Olive.

---

[32] Some of Olive's recipes were published in the book, "Recipes to Warm the Heart From The Heart of America, compiles by Cookbooks Unlimited, Loveland, Colorado and published by Cookbooks Publishers, Inc., Olathe, Kansas, 1993.

Stage 1: No Impairment/Normal Function

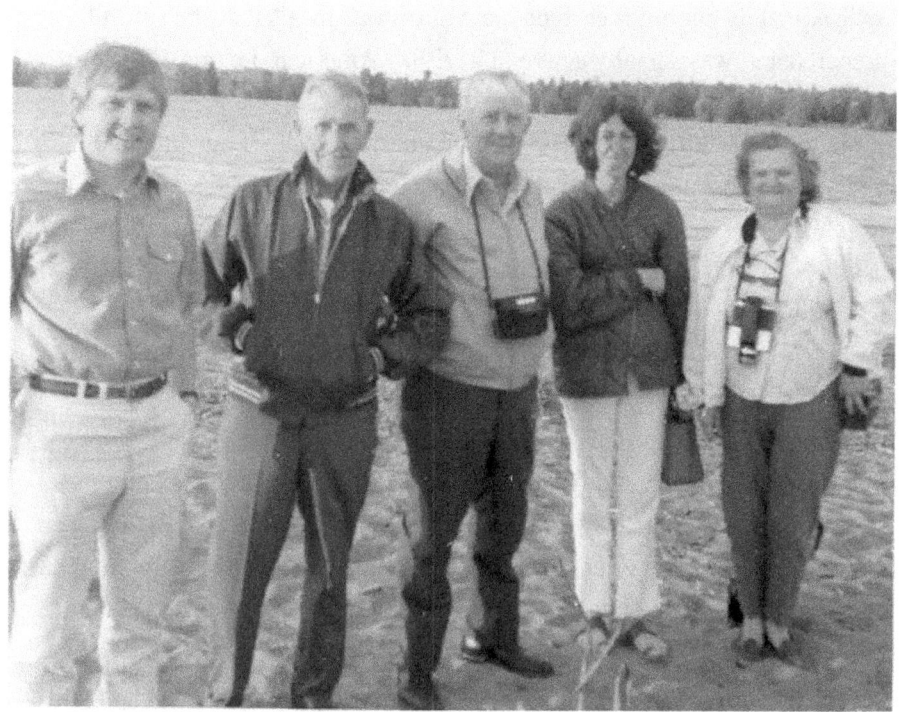

Figure 8: 1972 Parents & Uncle's Oregon Trip

Starting at age 54 in 1973, following her husband's sudden death, Olive's only heath concerns were cardiac problems resulting from the side effects of Rheumatic Fever and hypertension. Both were controlled by medication. Through the spring of 1998, Olive was an unimpaired individual who experienced no memory problems and none were evident to health care professional during medical interviews. Cardiac problems included atrial fibulation, hypertrophic cardiomyopathy and hypertension. Olive enjoyed her days doing genealogy research, oil painting (see art work in Figure 9: Rose Mauling on page 45, Figure 10: Oil Paintings on page 46 and Appendix J: Collage of Olive's Life on page 292), maintaining her home and lakeside cottage on nearby Lauderdale Lake, gardening, sewing, and visiting with friends and relatives. Olive liked to walk because she felt it was good for her heart and associated health. Typically, Olive walked at a brisk pace for approximately six miles each day, ate nutritious meals that she skillfully prepared and was socially active in TOPS,[33] American Legion Women's Auxiliary and interacted with a wealth of friends and relatives. For approximately thirty years, Olive maintained a weight of one hundred ten pounds, plus or minus three pounds, for which she received a TOPS award of which she was very proud. From 1940 through the mid nineties, Olive's height was 5' 2" but after the mid nineties Olive's height dropped below five feet probably due to osteoporosis.

I observed an undiagnosed potential neurological problem during the fifties when Olive would hesitate and not to be able to speak when the telephone rang or especially when she was suddenly surprised. Upon picking-up the phone, mother would hesitate for a few seconds before she was able to speak and answer the phone. I am not sure if this resulted from a neurological problem or another health issue. It was always a problem that concerned me. When I was in my teens, I felt sorry for mother that this speech problem existed. However, Olive did not allow this to hold her back in any way. She led an active life. Olive was always a very positive, upbeat person who enjoyed making people laugh and smile. When my dad told a joke, Olive had the loudest, most distinctive laugh of all.

Olive co-created a home environment where there was teamwork, seriousness about getting things done, as well as joy. My friend Sam described the Bublitz home best, "Your parent's home was a place of joy, laughter and general happiness where there was always something interesting going on. I enjoyed visiting your home even when you were away at college or in Vietnam."

---

[33] TOPS Club, Inc. is a non-profit charitable corporation based in Milwaukee, Wisconsin, USA, having members in chapters located worldwide, the majority of them in the United States and Canada. Its twofold objective is to sponsor research and foster support groups in human body weight control. Most members refer to the organization simply as "TOPS", an acronym for "Take Off Pounds Sensibly."

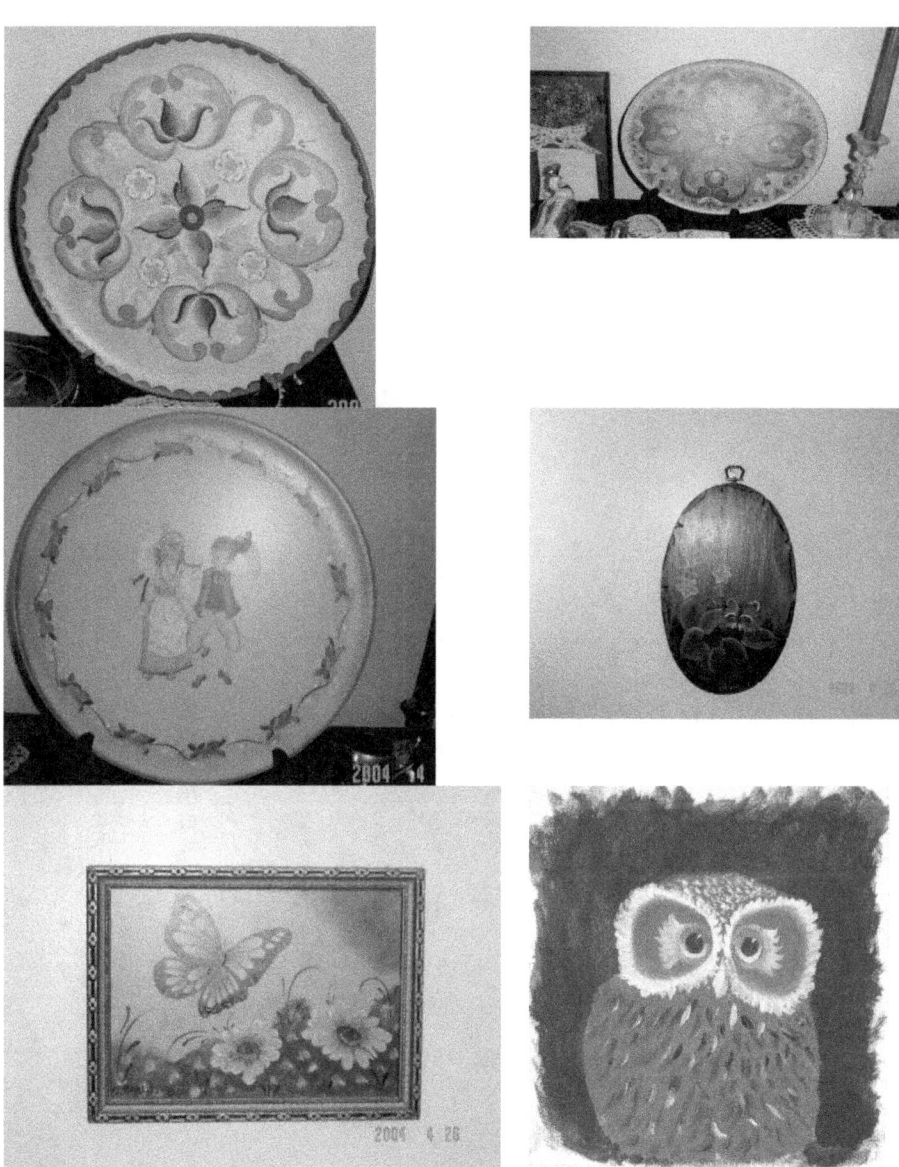

Figure 9: Rose Mauling Art Painted by Olive

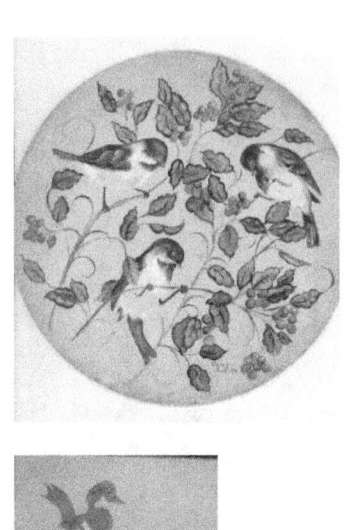

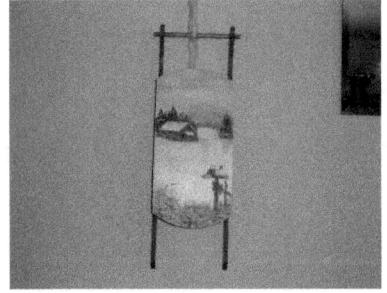

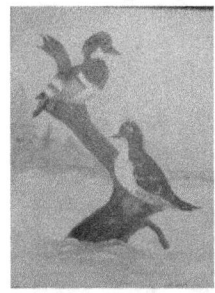

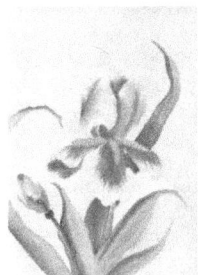

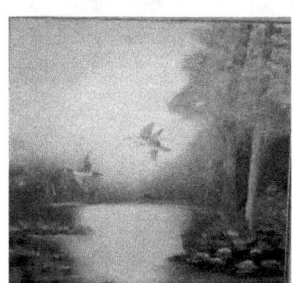

Figure 10: Oil Paintings by Olive

Stage 1: Enjoying Life

During this period, I would visit mother on weekends during frequent business trips to the East Coast or Midwest and spend a week during the summer visiting. Nearly every year Olive traveled by herself from her home in Wisconsin to my home on the West Coast to visit for a month. She would arrive in mid December and depart after her daughter-in-law's birthday in mid January. Her last visit traveling alone was in December 1995 through the January 1996 holidays. During this time, Olive's mental cognitive health seemed normal and we always enjoyed our visits. In between these visits, we would talk on the telephone weekly for fifteen to thirty minutes. Olive was visiting me when the Northridge earthquake occurred in Los Angeles on January 17, 1994. Upon returning to her home, the local paper where she worked part-time published an article on the front page describing her experience.

Throughout my entire life, one of the most important individuals and steadfast supporters in my life was always my mother. During my whole life whenever anything significant happened in my life, Olive would always get excited. Her happiness always magnified my own feelings and emotions about my success.

Stage 1: Recommendation to Immediate Family

Spend Quality Time Together

My advice at this stage is to prioritize, schedule and enjoy as much quality time together as possible. Life for all practical purposes is very short. Review photo albums to make sure the names of the people are noted, as well as the location and the date the photos were taken. Encourage genealogy research and documentation, obtain an oral history of the loved one's life, and take lots of pictures of family members, family friends and relatives, home, vacation places, church, etc.

Life Span Considerations

After reaching mid-life, one should seriously review a Life Span Table (see Figure 11 below). Make sure you understand the statistics on longevity so you are able to complete your life work and understand how long you and your loved ones are likely to live. The average life span today for someone born in 1960 who reaches sixty-five is seventy-eighty for a man and eighty-one for a woman.

Year	LIFE EXPECTANCY AT BIRTH		ADDITIONAL YEARS AFTER 65	
	Male	Female	Male	Female
1900	46.4	49.0	11.4	11.7
1920	54.5	56.3	11.8	12.3
1940	61.4	65.7	11.9	13.4
1960	66.7	73.2	12.9	15.9
1980	69.9	77.5	14.0	18.4
2000	73.2	79.7	15.8	19.3

Figure 11 Life Span Table[34]

Additionally, one should be aware of the fact that the number of Centenarians is increasing due to improvements in science, technology, medicine and care. Figure 12: Growth in Number of Centenarian on page 49 illustrates the growing number of people over the age one hundred.

Leading Causes of Death Statistics

Figure 13: Leading Causes of Death in U.S. on page 49 shows the leading causes of death beyond age 65 are heart disease, cancer and stroke. Surprising to many people is that at age 85, Alzheimer's disease ranks fourth. Alzheimer's is the fastest growing major cause of death due primarily to the fact that people are living longer. This is illustrated in Figure 14 on page 50 in the Los Angeles County Statistics report showing that Alzheimer's deaths

---

[34] Source of the data for this table is from the Office of the Chief Actuary, Social Security Administration.

grew by 220% from 1994 to 2003.

YEAR	2000	2010	2020	2030	2040	2050
Number of Centurions	72,000	131,000	214,000	324,000	447,000	834,000

Figure 12: Growth in Number of Centenarian[35]

Financially, the big difference between Alzheimer's and heart disease, cancer or stroke is that very little Alzheimer's care is covered by insurance. If a person has a heart attack and is taken to the hospital for heart surgery, a pacemaker or pacemaker- defibrillator implant, most of the expense will be covered by Medicare and the Medicare supplement. Likewise if a person has cancer and has radiation and/or chemotherapy, the expense will be covered by insurance. However, when a person develops Alzheimer's disease, unless

	65-74	65-74 Rank	75-84	75-84 Rank	> 85	> 85 Rank
All Causes	2,137.1		5,260.0		13,798.6	
Heart Disease	518.9	2	1,460.8	1	4,778.4	1
Cancer	742.7	1	1,274.8	2	1,637.7	2
Stroke	101.1	4	359.0	4	1,141.8	3
Respiratory	160.5	3	385.6	3	637.2	5
Diabetes	86.8	5	177.2	6	312.1	6
Alzheimer's	20.5	7	177.3	5	861.6	4
Accidents	46.3	6	106.1	7	279.5	7

Figure 13: Leading Causes of Death in U.S.[36]

[35] U.S. Bureau of Census, Current Population Reports, U.S. Government Printing Office, Washing, D.C.
[36] Rates on an annual basis are per 100,000 population in specific group. Source: National Vital Statistics Reports, Vol. 56, No. 10, April 24, 2008, National Center for Health Statistics (NCHS), U.S. Center for Disease Control (CDC).

CAUSE OF DEATH	1994	2003	PERCENT CHANGE
Heart Disease	276	196	-29.0
Stroke	63	51	-19.0
Lung Cancer	47	38	-19.1
Emphysema	35	34	-2.9
Pneumonia/Influenza	44	29	-34.1
Diabetes	20	26	30.0
Colorectal Cancer	20	17	-15.0
Alzheimer's	5	16	220.0
Breast Cancer	17	12	-29.4
Homicide	17	10	-41.2
HIV/AIDS	27	5	-81.5

Figure 14: Leading Cause of Death in Los Angeles County, 1994-2003[37]

the person has long-term care insurance which most people lack, the person is on their own. Most people with Alzheimer's end up spending every asset they accumulated during their entire lifetime to pay care expenses. The only way to protect your assets is to be impoverished and qualify for Medicaid Long Term Care. Many people are reluctant to impoverish themselves or a love one because of the low quality of care under Medicaid.

Determine End of Life Wishes

Ask the loved one what their wishes are in the case of an unexpected accident, illness or death. What would be their desires regarding a Health Directive? Whom would they want to assign Power of Attorney? In the case of death, how would they want their assets and personal property distributed?

---

[37] Source: Los Angeles County Public Health, Office of Health Assessment and Epidemiology.

Stage 1: No Impairment/Normal Function

Do they wish to have an autopsy for the benefit of their heir's health purposes and genealogy? Do they prefer a funeral or cremation? What mortuary, cemetery and graveside marker do they prefer?

Inventory Primary Assets & Personal Property

Suggest an inventory of all primary assets and personal property including photographs of the objects for potential insurance claims and long-term disposition. Several software packages are available for this purpose, for example, one is available from Intuit Inc..[38]

Discuss Impoverishment & Trust

An important discussion at this stage among the family is impoverishing the loved one. This maybe a sensitive issue unless there is substantial cash to afford the long-term cost of this potential disease. If the person is diagnosed with Alzheimer's, it will take time to position the person for Medicaid Benefits. Medicaid will conduct a three-year asset look back to determine qualification. As a result, it is important to get started with impoverishment as early as possible if it is felt that Medicaid Benefits will be needed to support the long-term care. This will reduce the financial burden on the family and position the person for Medicaid benefits. Most people prefer to have the fruits of their labor or assets go to their next of kin and let the government pay their medical expenses. Medicaid is a national government program that is administered by each state and has a variety of names. In California, the program is called Medical, in Wisconsin, Badgercare, etc. Under the Medicaid program, benefits may be received for in-home care or skilled nursing facilities.

Between age sixty-five and seventy-five consider placing all owned property in a Medicaid Qualifying Trust[39] and impoverishing yourself or loved one to protect the assets for disposition to the heirs thereby being able

---

[38] Quicken Home Inventory by Intuit Inc.

[39] For the latest information search the internet with the key phases, "Medicaid Qualifying Trust" or "Medicaid exempt trusts."

to qualify for government benefits through Medicaid. Currently, a person may own their own home, an automobile, bank deposits of not more than $2,000 and a monthly income not to exceed $1,911 to qualify for Medicaid Benefits (see Medicaid Long Term Care section, on page 120 for more details).

Select a Cemetery and Mortuary

It is also important to ask your love one who they would prefer you to use in the case of death for mortuary, church services and burial. If a funeral is held, find out who your loved one wants for pall bears and alternates. You should also choose a headstone together.

Philosophy on Death & Dying

Death is an important part of living. People, like flowers and nearly every living organism, go through a cycle of birth, growth, blooming, seed bearing, decline and death. However, in our Western Society today, people want to believe there is just prosperity and happiness. Unfortunately, that is not the reality of life. Life has its ups and downs. The most important thing is how you react to the various stimuli and the cycles of life. Alzheimer's disease is just one of those unfortunate periods for a loved one and their caregivers. How you respond to this journey determines if you grow or deteriorate from the experience. Alzheimer's disease will go full cycle and death is imminent.

Caregiving

Hold A Family Discussion on Caregiving & Decide How Family Members Share Responsibilities

As your loved one grows older, you and your family need to discuss caregiving. First, you need to discuss whose health and career will allow for the added responsibility. Next, you need to discuss the roles family members will contribute and who will assume primary responsibility. The primary caregiver, once selected and agreeing to the task, must begin a program to build physical and mental endurance to survive the task. First, if the person selected is not at or near the target weight for their age and height, I would highly recommend them setting a goal to adjust their weight to the target which is published by the National Institutes of Health.

Family members need to make sure the primary caregiver they select is healthy, is capable of the demanding caregiving task, and support their efforts with regular thoughtful physical assistance and communication.

Caregiver Health

This is the time for the person selected as the primary caregiver to get actively involved in building physical, mental, emotional and spiritual endurance in order to survive caregiving with their health intact.

Sabbatical to Care for Loved One - Then Resume Career Alternative

A common thought process of the children of an afflicted parent is, "I'll just take a sabbatical, care for mom and/or dad, or a spouse and then resume my career." The following are some examples of caregivers who followed this philosophy.

Friend Roger used this thought process when his father was diagnosed with Alzheimer's. Roger took a leave of absence from his station manager position with U.S. Airlines and moved three hundred miles to help his mother care for his father. The care for his father lasted three difficult years. A month later, Roger's mother fell, severely injuring her head and began to show similar symptoms and also was diagnosed with Alzheimer's disease. Roger continued to care for his mother for seven years. Because of all the stress and confusion of Alzheimer's, Roger began to lose his sight and today is legally blind. Later, after Roger's mother passed away, he visited his condominium for the first time in ten years. His former job was no longer available . . . and no other job was available.

A neighbor also used this philosophy to care for her mother. She took a sabbatical from her grade school teaching position with the Los Angeles Unified School District. Instead of lasting a year or two, the duration of the final three phases lasted eight stressful years. At the conclusion, her teaching credentials had expired and she had been away from her position so long that elementary school teaching was no longer an option.

Alzheimer's--What My Mother's Caregiving Taught Me

In my own case, prior to mother's diagnosis I had my best income year ever in the rapidly changing field of integrated circuit design software sales and marketing. After mother moved to California, I tried to continue to work from home, but it was not a viable option. Traveling out of town, which was necessary for success, was completely out of the question, even with a live-in caregiver and occasionally a second and third caregiver. In stage six of mother's disease I was diagnosed with cancer, had cancer surgery and a long recovery followed. This experience nearly took mother and I both down at the same time.

In summary, based on the cases that I have witnessed through the Alzheimer's Support Group and friends, once the afflicted enters stage five, the demands are so overwhelming it is difficult to accomplish anything else but care for your loved one. Taking a sabbatical to care for a parent or spouse and then planning to resume career is usually not a viable option.

Stage 2

Stage 2: Very Mild Cognitive Decline/Maybe Early Alzheimer's Sign

Typical at Stage 2: Individuals may feel as if they have memory lapses, especially in forgetting familiar words or names or the location of keys, eyeglasses or other everyday objects. Nevertheless, these problems are not evident during a medical examination or apparent to friends, family or co-workers.[40]

When you are in your 20s, you begin to lose brain cells a few at a time. Your body also starts to make less of the chemicals your brain cells need to work. The older you are, the more these changes can affect your memory. Aging may affect memory by changing the way the brain stores information and by making it harder to recall stored information. Your long-term memory is not usually affected by aging. However, your short term memory may be affected. For example, you may forget names of people you have met recently. These are normal changes.[41] Dementia causes many problems

---

[40] The Alzheimer Association Internet Site, September 2007, Alzheimer's Association National Office 225 N. Michigan Ave., Fl. 17, Chicago, IL 60601 or http://www.alz.org.

[41] Source: Written by familydoctor.org editorial staff. American Academy of Family Physicians, Reviewed/Updated: 12/06 Created: 01/96

for the person who suffers from it and for the person's family. Many of the problems are caused by memory loss. Some common signs of dementia are listed below. Not everyone who has dementia will have all of these signs:[42]

- Recent memory loss. All of us forget things for a while and then remember them later. People with dementia often forget things, but they never remember them. They might ask you the same question over and over, each time forgetting that you have already given them the answer. They will not even remember that they already asked the question.

- Difficulty performing familiar tasks. People who have dementia might cook a meal but forget to serve it. They might even forget that they cooked it.

- Problems with language. People who have dementia may forget simple words or use the wrong words. This makes it hard to understand what they want.

- Time and place disorientation. People who have dementia may get lost on their own street. They may forget how they got to a certain place and how to get back home.

- Poor judgment. Even a person who does not have dementia might get distracted. However, people who have dementia can forget simple things, like forgetting to put on a coat before going out in cold weather.

- Problems with abstract thinking. Anybody might have trouble balancing a checkbook, but people who have dementia may forget what the numbers are and what has to be done with them.

- Misplacing things. People who have dementia may put things in the wrong places. They might put an iron in the freezer or a wristwatch in the sugar bowl. Then they cannot find these things later.

---

[42] Source: Written by familydoctor.org editorial staff. Early Diagnosis of Dementia by KS Santacruz, M.D. and D Swagerty, M.D., M.P.H. (American Family Physician February 15, 2001, http://www.aafp.org/afp/20010215/703.html), Reviewed/Updated: 06/06, Created: 01/01.

Stage 2: Very Mild Cognitive Decline/Maybe Early Alzheimer's Sign

- Changes in mood. Everyone is moody at times, but people with dementia may have fast mood swings, going from calm to tears to anger in a few minutes.
- Personality changes. People who have dementia may have drastic changes in personality. They might become irritable, suspicious or fearful.
- Loss of initiative. People who have dementia may become passive. They might not want to go places or see other people.

Typically mild cognitive decline begins to be noticed when a person reaches the early sixties and is well underway by age eighty. Statistics indicate that at age sixty, five percent of the U.S. population has some degree of Alzheimer's disease and nearly half the people over eighty are faced with the illness.

Figure 15: Normal Age Related vs Alzheimer's Disease Memory Changes on page 58 is a table that should be used to help differentiate between someone with normal age related memory changes and one with Alzheimer's disease symptoms.

	A PERSON WITH NORMAL AGE-RELATED MEMORY CHANGES	A PERSON WITH ALZHEIMER'S DISEASE SYMPTOMS
Memory	Forgets part of an experience	Forget entire experience
	Often remembers later	Rarely remembers later
	Initially person can not find their keys or glasses, but later locates them later and carries out intended task	Person stands with keys or glasses in hand and is not sure what to do with them.
Following Instructions	Usually able to follow written/spoken directions	Gradually unable to follow written /spoken directions
Using Reminders	Usually able to use notes as reminders	Gradually unable to write legible notes or understand reminders
Caring for Self	Usually able to care for daily personal needs even with memory lapses (bathing, dressing, eating, taking medication, driving, etc.)	Gradually unable to care for daily personal needs even with memory lapses (bathing, dressing, eating, taking medication, driving, etc.)
Use of Household Appliances	Able to use TV controls and operate a Microwave Oven. Unlikely to leave kitchen range turned on.	Difficulty or inability to use TV controls or operate a Microwave Oven. Likely to leave kitchen range turned on.
Judgment	Able to make decisions	Seeks judgment of others
Tasking	Able to multi-task	Difficulty single tasking
Reaction time	Quick	Slow
Spatial Skills	Good Visual Discrimination	Impaired

Figure 15: Normal Age Related vs Alzheimer's Disease Memory Changes

Stage 2: Caregiving Begins

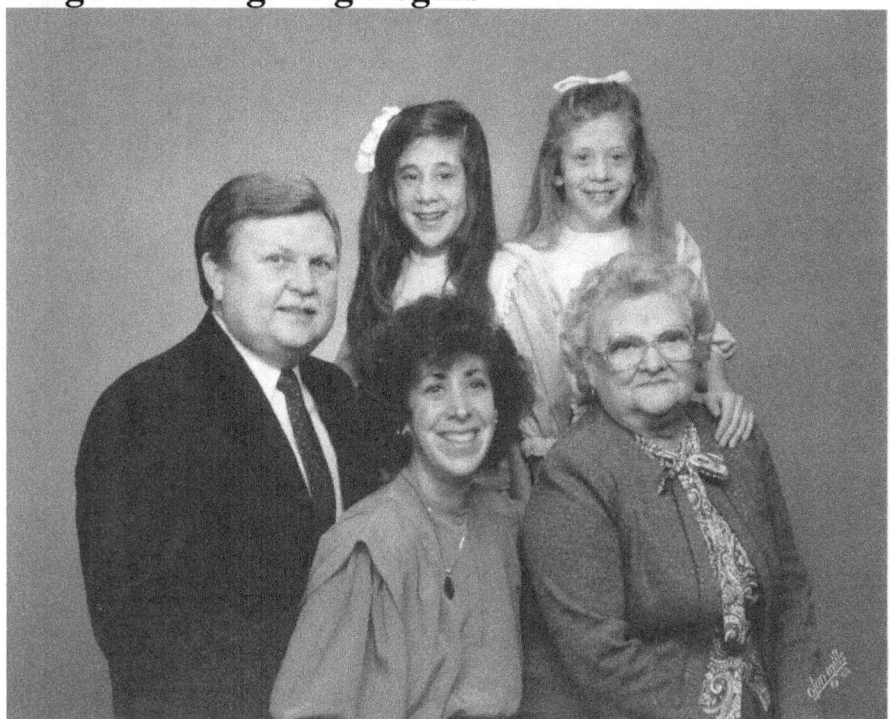

**Figure 16: Bob, Nina, Olive and Grandaughters, Aubrey and
Shelby, 1989**

Following the death of Olive's husband from a sudden and fatal heart
attack in November 1973 and especially after a ten-year relationship ended in
1987, mother began to show a mild cognitive decline. However, she
continued to be able to travel each Christmas to either Portland or Los
Angeles to spend a month with her son's family. Figure 16 is a photograph
from one of the many visits. Usually Olive stayed for her daughter-in-law's
birthday in mid January and returned to her home in Elkhorn, Wisconsin.
The travel day for this trip was usually a long twelve to fourteen hour day.
This is not a trivial trip for a person at any age. Olive would wake-up at five
o'clock, get dressed, finish packing and wait for a relative or friend to drive
her to the neighboring town of either Delevan or Janesville for an hour bus or

limousine ride to the O'Hare Airport Transportation Center. Arriving at O'Hare, Olive then had to locate a cargo cart and push her baggage a half mile to the United Airlines Terminal and check-in. Mother accomplished this long, strenuous task into her late seventies without a problem.

During the late nineteen eighties, Olive slowly ceased to be heavily involved with her genealogy research and oil painting, which she enjoyed. In the early nineteen nineties Olive stopped planting a vegetable garden behind her home because she said, "It was beginning to require too much of my declining energy." However, Olive continued to mow her lawn until the mid nineteen-nineties.

During the late nineteen-eighties through the mid nineteen-nineties, I think Olive began to feel as if she was experiencing memory lapses, especially in forgetting familiar words, names of places, relatives, friends and the location of keys, eyeglasses and other everyday objects. However, these problems were not evident during medical examinations or readily apparent to friends or other family members. In hindsight, during this phase the only thing that was unusual was mother's excessive talking on topics for long periods of time without any two-way communication with the intended listener. One can judge the degree of effectiveness of two-way communication by the degree of two-way interaction between the parties. Relative to this criterion, effective communication during this time seemed to decrease significantly.

Stage 2: Recommendation for Caregivers

Life today is usually very busy where both husband and wife work, may commute long distances to the site of their employment, spend time raising a family, do daily household chores and routine home maintenance. Because of this busy lifestyle, a person's awareness is overwhelmed by the immediate daily work and family routine. The reality is, people are so busy multi-tasking that there is little time to think; blurring ones awareness of what is going on around them. The result is that the declining health of aging parents or relatives goes unnoticed. My recommendation in this phase is to make sure the loved one is getting daily exercise, proper nutrition (Meals on Wheels is usually available at this stage) and make sure the person has significant daily social interaction. In addition, focus attention on the health of aging loved ones by making sure that every four years they have a routine physical exam which is paid for by Medicare. Also, make sure the loved one is routinely taking their medication on the specified schedule as well as taking a daily senior multivitamin.

Caregiving - The Beginning
Selecting & Building Patient Care Team

The document titled, Alzheimer Support Team on page 189 is an example of a chart you should begin to develop that describes your health care team with contact information.

Prioritize Quality Time Together

During Phase 2, you are going to begin to see memory changes in your loved one, especially beginning at age sixty-five. Use Figure 15: Normal Age Related vs Alzheimer's Disease Memory Changes on page 58 to help assess whether the changes are normal or Alzheimer related memory differences. Enjoy as much quality time together as possible.

End of Life Planning

It is important in this stage of life to have the following documents completed:

- Trust or Will
- Durable Power of Attorney
- Health Care Directive
- Do Not Resituate Order (DNR)
- Caregiver Essential Documents
- Final Arrangements

Examples of these documents are locate in Appendix A: Caregiver Essential Documents beginning on page 181 and Appendix B: Legal Document Examples beginning on page 199.

A copy of these documents, along with copies of property titles and insurance policies, should be kept in the home, distributed to the person who will assume Power of Attorney over the loved ones affairs and in a local bank lock box. The legal documents should be created with the assistance of a trusted attorney and/or computer software and be reviewed by a trust & estate attorney. At this time you may additionally want to check with National Academy of Elder Law Attorneys, Inc. (NAELA)[43] to locate an attorney familiar with Elder Law and begin to develop rapport with them.

---

[43] National Academy of Elder Law Attorneys, Inc. (NAELA)

Stage 3

Stage 3: Mild Cognitive Decline/Early-Stage Alzheimer

Typical at Stage 3: [44] Early-stage Alzheimer's can be diagnosed in some, but not all, individuals with these symptoms. Friends, family or co-workers begin to notice deficiencies. Problems with memory or concentration may be measurable in clinical testing or discernible during a detailed medical interview. Common difficulties include:

- Word or name finding problems become noticeable to family or close associates
- Decreased ability to remember names when introduced to new people
- Performance issues in social or work settings are noticeable to family, friends or co-workers
- Reading a passage and retaining very little of the content
- Losing or misplacing a valuable object
- Decline in ability to plan or organize

---

[44] The Alzheimer Association Internet Site, September 2007, Alzheimer's Association National Office 225 N. Michigan Ave., Fl. 17, Chicago, IL 60601 or http://www.alz.org.

Stage 3: Caregiving Continues

During 1996 Olive passed a Mini-Mental State Exam (MMSE) psychological tests (See description of test in Appendix C: Diagnosing Alzheimer's, Mini-mental state exam (MMSE), on page 241) at The Mayo Clinic in Rochester, MN prior to an electro-physiology study of Olive's heart. Prior to the study, the doctor discussed the possible need to perform heart surgery to correct an abnormal electrical conduction system. Luckily, the electro-physiology study indicated that surgery was not required. Instead, the doctors took Olive off all the medications she was taking except for hypertension medication. This was done because the doctors felt her problems might be occurring from being over medicated. The following year Olive experienced rapid arrhythmia problems several times and was hospitalized. During February 1997 we returned to The Mayo Clinic and she was placed in the hospital to see how she would tolerate a daily dose of 200 mg Amiodarone,[45] 120 mg of Dilitiazem,[46] and 20 mg of Lotensin.[47] Olive

---

[45] Amiodarone is an antiarrhythmic agent (medication used for irregular heart beat) used for various types of tachyarrhythmias (fast forms of irregular heart beat), both ventricular and supraventricular (atrial) arrhythmias. Discovered in 1961, it was not approved for use in the United States until 1985. Despite relatively common side-effects, it is used in arrhythmias that are otherwise difficult to treat with medication.
[46] Diltiazem is a member of the group of drugs known as benzothiazepines, which are a class of calcium channel blockers, used in the treatment of hypertension, angina pectoris, and some types of arrhythmia. It is a class 3 anti-anginal drug, and a class IV antiarrhythmic. It incites very minimal reflex sympathetic changes. Diltiazem is a potent vasodilator, increasing blood flow and variably decreasing the heart rate via strong depression of A-V node conduction. Its pharmacological activity is somewhat similar to verapamil. Diltiazem is metabolized by and acts as an inhibitor of the CYP3A4 enzyme. Diltiazem is relatively contraindicated in the presence of sick sinus syndrome, atrioventricular node conduction disturbances, bradycardia, impaired left ventricle function, peripheral artery occlusive disease, chronic obstructive pulmonary disease, and Prinzmetal's angina.
[47] Benazepril, brand name Lotensin, is a medication used to treat high blood pressure (hypertension), congestive heart failure, and chronic renal failure. Upon cleavage of its ester group by the liver, Benazepril is converted into its active form benazeprilat, a non-sulfhydryl angiotensin-converting enzyme (ACE) inhibitor.

was able to tolerate the medications without any side effects. She continued to take these medications after she returned home without any further need for hospitalization for arrhythmia problems. Prior to this time, a cousin was gracious to take mother to the hospital each time one of her arrhythmia incidents occurred.

An alternative to the medications during the 1990s was a combined pacemaker-defibrillator. However, due to its size it would have to be worn externally on a belt attached to her body. Mother said she would not wear one because of the size and inconvenience. During early 2000, a combination implantable pacemaker-defibrillator came on the market. The U.S. Vice President, Cheney, was one of the first recipients to receive an implantable miniaturized silver dollar size version of this device.

Before I returned to California on this trip in late February 1997, mother and I went to the grocery store. Since it would be difficult for mother to get to the store during the long, severe Wisconsin winter, I bought her a variety of meats: chicken legs, spare ribs and some cuts of beef that she enjoyed. I froze the meat and also froze some fresh fish which I caught through the ice from a neighboring lake. Olive always enjoyed eating fish from the local lakes.

At this time, mother continued to walk daily. However, when we walked at the lake, Olive had difficulty navigating the hills. In addition, she began to spend more time looking at the ground in front of her instead of enjoying the scenery during the walk.

Stage 3: Recommendation for Caregivers

At this stage, it is essential to discuss who is going to be the primary caregiver. I hope that this decision has already been made and all the legal documents are in order.

Financing Care

Financing Alzheimer's care becomes a problem for nearly every family caring for a loved one because of the long duration of the illness and stress of the care. In the case of elderly couples, it is common for them to sell their family home to generate cash to pay for the care of a loved one afflicted with Alzheimer's disease. Once the home is sold, the proceeds are usually used to pay for a board and care home while the other spouse downsizes to a condominium or apartment to free up needed cash. In the case of a child caring for a parent, it is common for one to move in with the other. In the end, the care will use up nearly every asset available. The cost of Alzheimer's patient care is estimated at over a half million dollars per person during stages five through seven. As a result of the long duration of the care, cost of care and hardship on immediate families, it has turned into a national crisis because of the vast number of new cases every week.

This is the reason it is so necessary for a family to begin impoverishing the loved one as soon as the disease has been diagnosed. When the person is impoverished and assets are no longer available to support the disease, Medicaid Long Term Care (LTC) will take over payment of expenses for in-home care. As the disease progresses, Medicaid LTC will also pay for the care in a skilled nursing facility once the person is impoverished.

End of Life Plans Complete

It is important in this stage of life to have the following documents completed and in a single location for quick access:

- Durable Power of Attorney for Financial Affairs that is current and notarized
- Property Titles & Insurance are up to date
- Trust or Will
- Asset inventory of all personal property owned by the person with Alzheimer's Disease
- Advanced Health Care Directive that is current and notarized
- Do Not Resituate Order (DNR), which is current and notarized, to go into effect during phase six or seven as Alzheimer's disease progresses
- Complete Personal Balance Sheet and Income & Expense Report
- "Free" Annual Credit Report to see if there are any unexpected debts or claims

Impoverishment should be started at this stage and complete not later than early stage five.

Additionally, build a contact list including names, addresses and phone numbers of friends and relatives so you will be able to keep them up to date on health status, mail them holiday cards and when appropriate, notify them of funeral arrangements.

Place a High Priority on Quality Time Together

Lastly, and most importantly in Stage three, is to spend as much quality time as possible with your loved one. Go walking together, enjoy coffee or meals together, go to the movies, a concert or play, etc. Reminisce about the past; consider doing an oral history that is recorded on a DVD and also transcribed in print form.

Stage 4

Stage 4: Moderate Cognitive Decline/Mild or Early-Stage Alzheimer

Typical at Stage 4:[48] a careful medical interview by a neurologist and a neuropsychologist will detect clear-cut deficiencies in the following areas:

- Decreased knowledge of recent occasions or current events
- Impaired ability to perform challenging mental arithmetic-for example, to count backward from 75 by 7s
- Decreased capacity to perform complex tasks, such as planning dinner for guests, paying bills and managing finances
- Reduced memory of personal history
- The affected individual may seem subdued and withdrawn, especially in socially or mentally challenging situations

---

[48] The Alzheimer Association Internet Site, September 2007, Alzheimer's Association National Office 225 N. Michigan Ave., Fl. 17, Chicago, IL 60601 or http://www.alz.org.

Stage 4: Moderate Cognitive Decline/Mild or Early-Stage Alzheimer

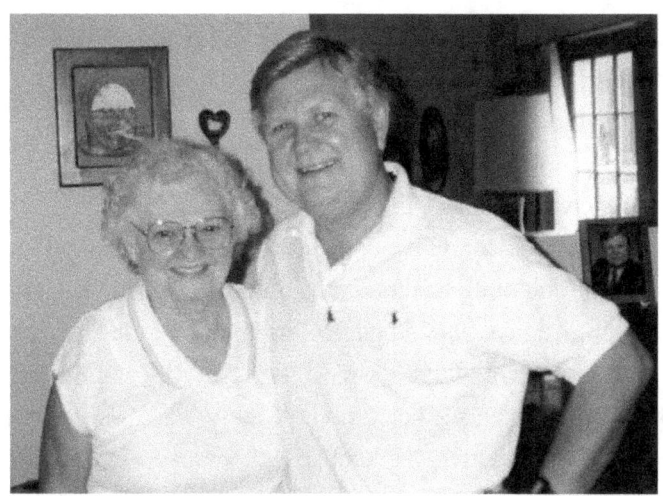

Figure 17: Olive & Her Son, Bob, August 1998

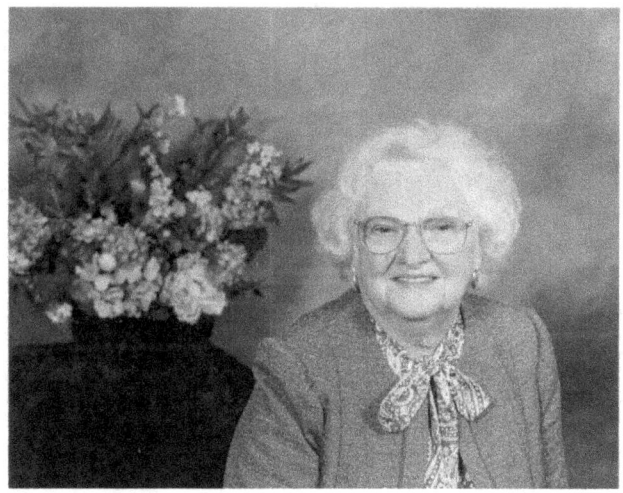

Figure 18: Olive, November 1999

Stage 4: Caregiving Requires More Time

During the spring 1998, mother fell after lunch while walking with friends from a restaurant to a theater to see a play. When Olive tripped and fell, she suffered a concussion and was taken to the hospital in Fort Atkinson, Wisconsin. A few days later Olive was released and recovered at home.

Because of the accident, Olive experienced double vision and rarely left her home for a period of eighteen months until early 2000. Figure 17: Olive & Her Son, Bob, August 1998 on page 69 is a photograph taken three or four months after the accident. I believe if you look closely at mother's eyes and facial expression, you can see her vision difficulty and discomfort from the accident. In Figure 18: Olive, November 1999 on page 75 it appears Olive's overall health has improved since the accident. This picture was taken for the church's Annual Financial Report and Member Directory. It is interesting that Olive never mentioned or sent me a copy of this beautiful portrait. Maybe it was because she was forgetful at the time. Instead, I found the picture when I was preparing Olive's home for sale.

The 1998 accident was likely the beginning of the Alzheimer's that can be diagnosed in some, but not all individuals. During 1999 and 2000, Olive's friends and family began to notice forgetfulness and difficulties with simple tasks as well as other deficiencies. Problems with memory or concentration may have been measurable in clinical testing or discernible during a detailed medical interview, but one was not conducted at this time. Friends and family members however began to notice Olive's difficulty operating her microwave, television remote controls and keeping track of days of the week. A friend in Las Vegas at this time sent Olive an elaborately hand painted calendar which Olive used to keep track of the day of the week by moving the dates to the day of the appropriate week.

During August 2001, I returned to Wisconsin to do some maintenance on mother's home and nearby lakeside cottage. Also at this time mother was having problems with a neighbor whose children allegedly during the previous four years smashed every window out of the factory building Olive

Stage 4: Moderate Cognitive Decline/Mild or Early-Stage Alzheimer

owned. The factory building was located behind the neighbor's house. The neighbor often had overnight female guests visit her home. This bothered mother as well as many of her small town neighbors. The woman's oldest son committed suicide in his mother's garage which was located next to mother's house. To make things even more stressful, when I was home during August, the neighbor instigated a "Building Condemnation Order" on the factory building with the city of Elkhorn. Two police officers arrived on noisy motorcycles to deliver the "Condemnation Order." The incident caused concern for me because I thought mother might have a heart attack from all the noise and stress. Mother immediately turned to the police officers and said, "Why that son of a bitch neighbor of mine, she is up to it again." Olive then turned and looked at the neighbor's house to see if she was looking out the window. Immediately I called an attorney of a mutual friend who arrived at the house within an hour. Upon arrival, we sat down and discussed the situation and alternatives to resolve the matter. The following day I drove to the city sheriff's office and met with the police chief. I indicated mother had a serious coronary condition and I was surprised that she did not have a heart attack the previous day by the noisy, disruptive way the Condemnation Order was delivered by two police officers riding motorcycles. The police chief listened to my concerns and then showed me a one inch thick, three ring binder of reports with background information on the neighbor. He said, "I am aware of the problem in the neighborhood." I asked him to address any further communication to myself, which he agreed. Later I met with the building inspector regarding the same subject. To resolve the matter it took the attorney a year and over fifty thousand dollars to resolve the dispute.

During September 2001, I took mother to The Mayo Clinic primarily for a routine cardiac check-up, urinary and digestive tract analysis and vision testing. Mother complained that her vision had declined. Olive also thought she had a potential urinary or digestive tract problem that was causing her to frequently use the bathroom. On the way to The Mayo Clinic, we stopped at a gas station. Inside the gas station, I observed mother walking out of the bathroom and then turning around and walking back into the bathroom four times in less than ten minutes. The Mayo Clinic testing took approximately two weeks. During this time, a general physical and lab tests were conducted plus additional testing of her heart, vision, urinary & digestives tract, hearing and a mammogram. The urinary and digestives system testing included a digestive nuclear transport study which did not reveal any problem. The vision testing also did not reveal a need for cataract surgery. Olive's local ophthalmologist was encouraging her to buy new eyeglasses and consider cataract surgery. The gastroenterologists we met with regarding her need to frequently use the bathroom, mentioned to me in private that the problem might be related to an aging mental condition. However, a potential mental problem was not investigated at this time. At the end of the testing, we met with the cardiologist for a final consultation. The cardiologist said, "Olive's heart problems had not progressed and there were no other problems evident that required medical attention." We all felt this was good news. The meeting with the cardiologist was held over lunch since she had to cancel our scheduled morning meeting for an emergency. Afterward, the female doctor gave mother a big hug and we returned to Olive's home.

On this visit I did some yard work and tree trimming at mother's home in Elkhorn. I noticed that Olive's meals were simpler than in the past. She would wake up in the morning at seven, eat cereal or toast for breakfast and drink a cup coffee. At noon, she would eat a sandwich for lunch. Dinners were simple and there seemed to be a reluctance to prepare the elaborate meals of the past. Each afternoon or early evening we went for a six-mile walk around town that was part of mother daily routine. We visited several friends and relatives. My close cousin Don and his wife June told me in private that they noticed mother having difficulties with simple tasks. For example, the previous Thanksgiving and Christmas they invited mother to their home for the Holidays. Olive prepared the pistachio salad that had become Olive's traditional contribution for their family dinners. Preparation of the salad simply involved opening a box of pistachio Jell-O powder, mixing it with hot water, chilling the mixture, then adding marshmallows and

Stage 4: Moderate Cognitive Decline/Mild or Early-Stage Alzheimer

whipped cream before it is served. June said Olive kept calling her repeatedly to make sure she was making it properly. On one occasion upon arrival at Don and June's home, the pistachio salad was runny. Mother either did not make it correctly or took it out of the refrigerator too early.

June later told me about an incident involving her own mother. One evening June's mother called her daughter Lucile and said, "Lucile, come over quickly, people have come up from the Mississippi river and are sitting in the trees around the house." June said her sister got in her car and drove swiftly to her mother's home. When Lucile arrived, her mother met her at the front door and they immediately walked to a back room of the house where her mother said emotionally, "See them, they are sitting in the trees with lanterns." Lucile in complete disbelief did not see anything in the trees, but invited her mother to her home for a few days. After returning to her mother's home a couple of days later, Lucile realized that the alleged people and lanterns in the trees were probably fireflies. When June's mother returned to her home a couple of days later, she had forgotten the episode. Shortly after the incident, June's mother was diagnosed with dementia and placed in a home.

Don related a similar situation with his mother, as she grew elderly. Don's mother was cared for by a live-in caregiver. The caregiver took many of his mother's jewelry pieces and other valuable personal items; sadly not an uncommon problem. Eventually his mother had to be placed in a nursing home. However, one Saturday morning prior to her admittance to the nursing home Don visited his mother. During his visit as they were enjoying conversation over a cup of coffee, his mother said, "Don, see that hole over there under the cabinets? A mouse keeps coming out of that hole, stands-up on his back legs and laughs at me." In disbelief, Don said, "Oh! Really? His mother repeated the story during several later visits. Finally one morning when she made the comment, Don went over to where the mouse was allegedly standing, stomped on him, held the mouse up by the tail and said, "See mom, he's not going to bother you any more" and pretended to flush the mouse down the toilet. This ended his mother's concerns with the mouse and she never talked about it again.

One evening in the autumn of 2001 when my mother and I were staying at the lake, the weather turned cold. When I turned on the heat, Olive got panicky and said, "Turn off the heat, I don't have the money to pay for the gas." Another time I went for a walk in the evening. When I returned mother was crying. I asked mother, "Why are you crying?" Olive said, "You know, I don't like to be out here alone by myself when it is dark. I get scared. What if something happens to me, how would I get help?" During this time, my cousin Don and June looked after mother. They said that she was becoming very forgetful. On two occasions at the lake during September 2001, mother made dinners with the assistance of her recipe cards for cousins Elmer and then a week later for Larry and Lana without any apparent difficulty. Each time it was the same exact dinner menu: country style pork ribs, sauerkraut, onions, carrots and potatoes. In the second case, prior to their visit, I mentioned to my cousins Lana and Larry that mother was becoming very forgetful. At the end of their evening visit, I walked them to their car. Lana turned to me after entering the vehicle, rolled down her window and said, "Bob, you have nothing to worry about. From my conversation with Olive tonight, your mother's mind is as sharp as a tack." This example illustrates how mother was able to rise up to the occasion for special events and seem very normal. The next day she would have difficulty with simple tasks like dressing herself. This is a common occurrence as Alzheimer's disease progresses.

During this time, we also drove to Milwaukee to meet Olive's sister Betty and her daughter Karen and son-in-law Jim. A picture from the trip is illustrated in Figure 19 on page 75. We enjoyed lunch together at a restaurant in a Milwaukee suburb and then took pictures of Olive and her sister Betty. Mother was thrilled to be able to visit her sister and they talked extensively, smiled frequently and enjoyed the outing. Later in 2008, Olive's sister Betty was not feeling good, complaining of a headache and dizziness and was taken to a local hospital where she died of a sudden, unexpected brain aneurysm on September 17, 2008 two days before her eighty-fifth

Stage 4: Moderate Cognitive Decline/Mild or Early-Stage Alzheimer

birthday.

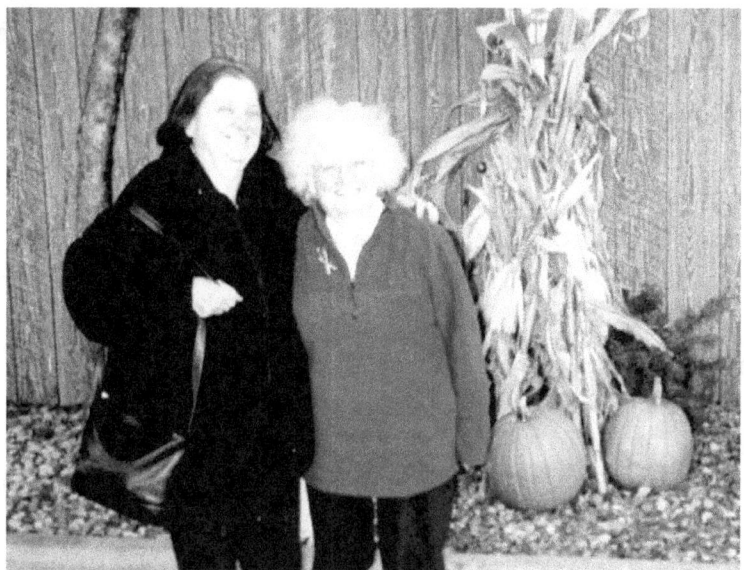

Figure 19: Olive and her Sister, Betty, Milwaukee, WI, October 2001

During this time, a neighbor across the street was helping mother with her shopping needs. Additionally, each evening mother would turn a front door light on around nine o'clock and the neighbor would reciprocate. Then mother would turn her light off at ten and the neighbor would do the same. This indicated to each other that everything was ok. Also at this time another friend, who belonged to the same church as mother and whose brother had worked for my father, helped Olive pay her bills, handle her taxes and other financial matters. Handwriting changed during this stage and sometimes Olive would begin to write a check and then mark it "void." She would often do this several times. Other times she would have difficulty writing, even with a line as a guide. Her handwriting would often drift above the line or migrate below the line. Notes that she made became illegible.

Beginning in stage four, two women from the church began visiting mother weekly in the afternoon. They would begin by sharing newspaper clippings and then discuss local news and church events. The church pastor also visited mother monthly. He would often read bible scriptures to satisfy Olive's spiritual needs, give her communion occasionally and discuss church and member's activities. During this time, Olive would sit in a recliner with her legs crossed under her like a young girl. She started sitting in this position around 2000.

During 2001, Olive continued to live alone. In hindsight, I believe that at this stage a full neuro-psychological testing would have detected likely Alzheimer's disease. Mother was always concerned about not worrying her son about her health. Instead, she kept mental difficulties to herself and a few trusted friends. Olive was able to mask many of her problems by being very organized and she possessed extremely good social skills. If anyone asked Olive a question, she would reply, "Well, what do you think?" Then she would repeat what the person had told her. In hindsight I feel Olive exhibited all the symptoms listed above in Stage Four Alzheimer disease during 2001.

A few weeks after this visit I returned to my home in Los Angeles feeling comfortable that mother could take care of herself, repairs on and around the house had been completed and we had a successful trip to The Mayo Clinic where they did not find anything of concern with Olive's health. At the time, I thought maybe I was overly concerned about mother's declining health condition.

Before Christmas 2001, my friend Kirt called and asked if my mother was ok. I said, "I think so, I talked to her the last two weekends and she sounded ok, but why do you ask?" Kirt said," I have driven by your house several times in the last two weeks when it has snowed almost continuously and I don't see any human footprints in the snow or car tracks. Today, I stopped by the house with a poinsettia for your mother and she did not come to the door. As I walked around the house, she finally came to the door and was excited by the Christmas present." In late December when I arrived at the house, mother proudly pointed out the beautiful plant that Kirt had personally delivered to mother. I feel at the time I was blinded by the career activity

Stage 4: Moderate Cognitive Decline/Mild or Early-Stage Alzheimer

going on in my life and concern for two daughters in college.

Stage 4: Recommendation for Caregivers

At Stage 4, or typically between the ages of 75 and 82, life begins to become very stressful for seniors. They have experienced the death of many friends and relatives, many surviving ones face serious illness, their circle of friends becomes smaller, financial problems may intensify and they experience loneliness. This is a time to be particularly observant of a loved one's behavior. If you are young and do not have an aging parent or grandparent, this may be the time to begin a friendship with a senior to be enlightened by what you will face when you grow old and to help the elderly person. The rewards will be mutually satisfying.

Consider Full Neuro-psychological Testing

If the person is showing symptoms of Alzheimer's described in Figure 15: Normal Age Related vs Alzheimer's Disease Memory Changes on page 58 it is time to consider Full Neuro-psychological Testing as described in Appendix C: Diagnosing Alzheimer's, on page 239.

Decision to Stop Driving

The decision to stop driving a car is usually the first major decision that is difficult for an afflicted person to handle. It is difficult because it is the first decision that limits the person's freedom and independence. However, it is necessary to protect the safety of the loved one, the driver of other vehicles and pedestrians along the road. Mother made this decision by herself without any discussion after her auto accident November 2001.

Reluctance to make this decision may result in the afflicted person getting on the freeway, getting lost and several hours later calling to be picked-up or having law enforcement involved. Worse yet is the high potential for an accident with other vehicles or pedestrians. To help facilitate this decision a driver's reality checklist is included on page 184.

Very High Priority on Quality Time Together

During this phase, you want to spend as much quality time together as possible. This is one of the final stages for good two-way communication while your loved one is lucid. Expect chaos and unpredictability in the next stage of the disease.

Denial

The biggest problem that must be dealt with in this phase is denial. One day the person seems normal, the next day the person is not able to tie their shoes, may put on two different shoes or be unable to dress themselves or complete other simple tasks. Mother kept index cards with notes, inventory of food items and a contact information list for friends and relatives. During the transition from this phase into the next, her handwriting drifted off a straight line and started to become illegible. When mother knew that someone was scheduled for a visit, she seemed to be able to rise up to the occasion and seem very normal. Some friends even said, "Bob, you worry too much. Your mother's mind is as sharp as a tack." Regarding things that happened way back in the past, Olive was able to remember them without difficulty. However, when it came to asking her what she did the day before or the week before, Olive could hardly remember anything. This is the stage to schedule a full neuropsychological testing as described in Appendix C: Diagnosing Alzheimer's, on page 239. Ideally it should be at one of the approximately thirty federally-funded Alzheimer's Disease Centers (ADCs) enacted by an Act of Congress (Public Health Service Act, section 445) in 1984. An ADC directory is listed by state in Appendix D: Alzheimer Disease Research Centers, beginning on page 259. At these centers, you can be confident that qualified personnel are available to make a thorough, quality assessment.

The Consequence of Denial

The consequences of denial of not getting a diagnosis when indications warrant one, procrastination or failure to get personal matters in order and do the proper planning will result in complete chaos. Additionally, it will jeopardize the health of the primary caregiver and other family members. The family assets that the afflicted one worked so hard to accumulate and hoped to pass on to their heirs could be completely depleted.

Stage 4: Moderate Cognitive Decline/Mild or Early-Stage Alzheimer

Consider Enrollment in "Meals-on-Wheels"

Eating regular breakfast, lunch and dinner meals is very important in this stage. This insures that the lack of nourishment is not contributing to the health condition. Meals-on-Wheels is available to the elderly either free of charge or for a small fee by calling a local representative. I would highly recommend the services in stages four and five.

Caregiver Signing of Documents

Caregivers should be cautious when signing documents for an Alzheimer's patient. You will want to check with an elder law attorney during the early stage of Alzheimer's disease to understand the financial liability you might incur in the state where the Alzheimer's patient will live during the three late stages. In some states if you sign your name followed by "for (the Alzheimer's patient name)," your liability is different than simply signing only your own signature. "Signing for" in some states protects the caregiver from financial liability if the estate of the Alzheimer's patient runs out of assets. Be sure to consult with your elder law attorney during the early stages of the disease to understand this issue because it could save you hundreds of thousands of dollars. Also, not knowing the legalities could negatively affect your credit.

Stage 5

Stage 5: Moderately Severe Cognitive Decline/Early-Stage Alzheimer's

Typical at Stage 5:[49] major gaps in memory and deficits in cognitive function emerge. Some assistance with day-to-day activities becomes essential. At this stage, individuals may:

- Be unable during a medical interview to recall such important details as their current address, their telephone number or the name of the college or high school from which they graduated
- Become confused about where they are or about the date, day of the week or season
- Have trouble with less challenging mental arithmetic, for example, counting backward from 40 by 4s or from 20 by 2s
- Need help choosing proper clothing for the season or the occasion
- Usually retain substantial knowledge about themselves and know their own name and the names of their spouse or children
- Usually require no assistance with eating or using the toilet

---

[49] The Alzheimer Association Internet Site, September 2007, Alzheimer's Association National Office 225 N. Michigan Ave., Fl. 17, Chicago, IL 60601 or http://www.alz.org.

Stage 5: Moderately Severe Cognitive Decline/Early-Stage Alzheimer's

Brain Atrophy and Alzheimer's Disease

Figure 20: Brain Atrophy and Alzheimer's on page 82, shows four magnetic resonance images (MRI) of four different people with differently sized and shaped brains. The widening grooves and fissures of the cerebral cortex indicate progressively severe brain atrophy and loss of brain mass from normal to mild Alzheimer's, moderate Alzheimer's and severe Alzheimer's.

Diagnosis

During November 2001, Olive was involved in an auto accident and failed a mental test at her primary local family doctor's office. Olive's primary physician in Elkhorn recommended a brain MRI to see if there was brain injury from the auto accident.

In early January 2002, I took a flight from my home in the Los Angeles area to mother's home in the Midwest. On the first evening home, mother gave me an unopened letter from the police department. Mother said, "Here Bob, I think this is the accident report, will you please open the letter and read it to me." Before I could open the envelope, mother said she was not at fault in the accident. Mother stated, "The vehicle that hit me was traveling over the speed limit and I did not see the vehicle when I drove off from the stop sign and the vehicle hit my Buick broadside." She continued, "The driver even apologized to me at the scene of the accident for traveling over the speed limit." According to mother, at the scene of the accident the other driver also said, "I'm sorry, I didn't see you, the accident is my fault." The accident report said, "Olive was at fault." Usually a driver that hits another vehicle is at fault since a person is supposed to have their vehicle under control at all times. This was not the case in this accident. To me this was the second example of several cases I witnessed of someone taking advantage of an elderly person, especially when a person broadsides another vehicle, this time by an official city employee.

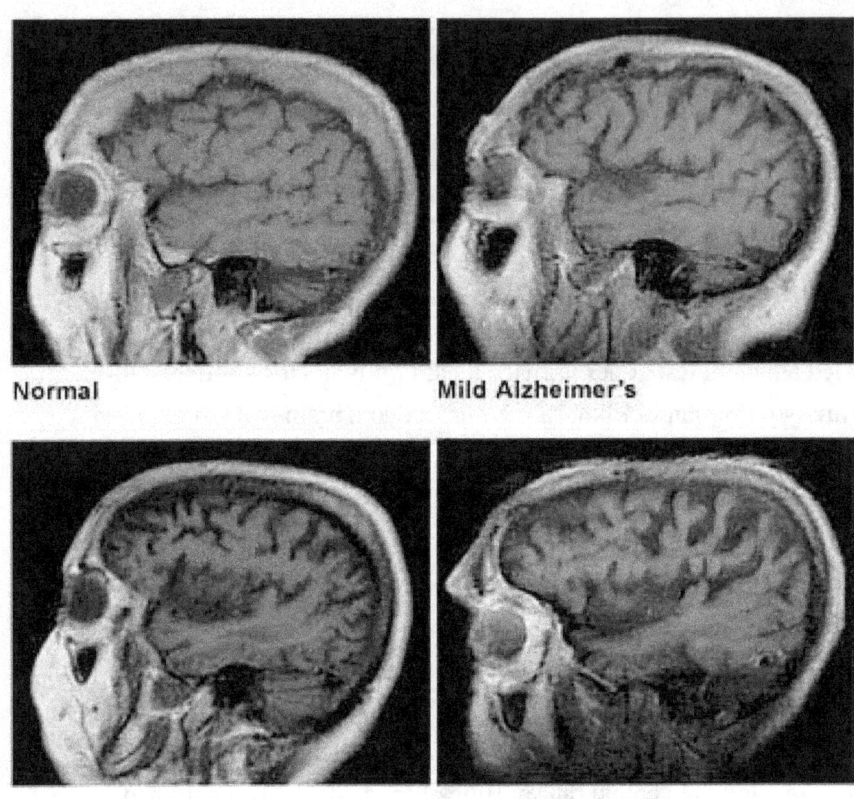

Normal

Mild Alzheimer's

Moderate Alzheimer's

Severe Alzheimer's

Figure 20: Brain Atrophy and Alzheimer's[50]

---

[50] The Mayo Clinic, Rochester, MN or
http://www.mayoclinic.com/health/medical/MO2896.

Stage 5: Moderately Severe Cognitive Decline/Early-Stage Alzheimer's

Sunday, January 20, 2002, we drove in Olive's red 91 Buick Skylark, of which she was so proud, to The Mayo Clinic three hundred miles away. The following week, a MRI was performed on mother's brain and pelvic area. Following the MRI, full neuropsychological testing was performed. The good news from the tests was, "there was no brain injury from the accident." The bad news was that Olive had a fairly advanced case of Alzheimer's disease, osteoporosis and degenerative joint disease and would no longer be able to live alone.

The MRI from The Mayo Clinic showed, "no acute lesions. The amount of white matter change was minimal. There was prominent cerebral atrophy and ventricular enlargement but the doctor indicated she does not have hydrocephalus (see Figure 20: Brain Atrophy and Alzheimer's on page 82). Hippocampus atrophy was quite striking." The neurologist comments after the neuropsychological tests indicated the following, "I believe that she probably had an underlying dementing illness, probably Alzheimer's disease, for some time that was well compensated. Then with her minor motor vehicle accident, which I believed caused no significant brain injury, it upset her usual scheme of activities and made her seem more confused and disabled her compensatory mechanism. In addition, her relative social isolation by not being able to drive may have exacerbated the problem further. If this hypothesis is correct, then she is unlikely to show any substantial improvement over time but neither is she likely to worsen dramatically either. This would mean that Olive's living situation at the present time is probably not satisfactory and she would need to be in a more stable living situation, probably with her son out where he lives in Los Angeles. The alternative hypothesis is that she has a more rapidly progressive dementing illness and it could worsen dramatically." See Appendix F: Olive's Clinical Diagnosis, 272 for the complete report.

Decision to Change Living Arrangement

Upon returning to Olive's home from The Mayo Clinic in January 2002, mother willingly decided to join me in California and live in my home. We spent the late summer and early fall of 2002 in Wisconsin. When the time came to leave for California in late fall 2002, mother started to question her decision. After several delays and discussions with friends and relatives, we left for California. This was a very difficult time for mother. I believe she knew her health was rapidly deteriorating and fought the logical decision that to live in California was in her best interest. Perhaps mother knew that she would never again see the home that she loved and that held so many memories accumulated over the sixty years she had lived there.

Stage 5: Caregiving Intensifies - Physically & Emotionally Demanding & Chaotic at Times

Following the trip to The Mayo Clinic during January 2002, we returned to mother's home and spent approximately two weeks before we departed for California. The first morning at mother's home while we were sitting in the living room drinking coffee, mother asked me to read the report from The Mayo Clinic to her again. This was probably the fourth or fifth time I read the summary to mother. During the reading, mother listened but I do not think she could comprehend the seriousness of the report. At the end of the reading mother turned to me and said, "So what are you going to do with me?" I said, "Mother, it depends on what you would like to do?" Mother said, "I don't care as long as there are people around. I have been very lonely."

At this point, Olive moved to my home in California, continued to walk everyday, sometimes even alone. During this time, major gaps in memory and deficits in cognitive function emerged. Olive required some assistance with day-to-day activities but was still fairly independent.

During the spring of 2002, mother and I attended Tai Chi classes for an hour on Tuesdays and Thursdays. In April 2002, we toured Senior Concerns, a day care facility for elderly people with dementia. When we returned to the car, mother turned to me and said, "Bob, I don't think this place or their programs would be good for me . . . why, I still have my marbles." During

Stage 5: Moderately Severe Cognitive Decline/Early-Stage Alzheimer's

August 2002, Mother started attending programs at Senior Concerns and enjoyed every day. Figure 21 on page 86, shows a typical Senior Concerns monthly activity calendar. Figure 22 on page 87, displays some of the creative projects mother made at Senior Concerns. When you compare Olive's previous rose mauling and art to the craft projects at the Senior Concern, you can see the decline in the complexity and creativity of her artistic ability. On several occasion I joined mother, sometimes alone or with one of my daughters for events like Hawaiian Days, Dog Fridays and other special occasions.

Monday	Tuesday	Wednesday	Thursday	Friday
AUGUST Birthdays 9 George/Ann C. 18 Ed G. 24 Afton P. 25 Leonard K. 26 Pete N.	**Dining Room Hours** Morning Snack 8:30 Lunch 11:30 Afternoon Snack 2:30	**Extended Hours** Monday - Friday 7:30 am - 9:00 am 3:00 pm - 5:30 pm 2nd & 4th Sat 11 am-4 pm	Shabbat 1st and 3rd Fridays Christian Life 4th Tuesday Sam's Dogs Visit Every Friday Podiatry Appointments 8/29	**1** 9:00 Coffee Klatch & Puzzles 9:30 News & Discussion 10:00 Anna's Sewing Bee 10:00 Bob's Band 11:00 Easy Exercise with Stephanie 1:00 Staff Talent Show 2:00 Bingo Time 3:00 Snacks and say goodbye
4 Coast Guard Day 9:00 Coffee Klatch & Puzzles 9:30 News & Discussion 10:00 Bhojo Entertains 10:00 Crafts Club with Anna 11:00 Stretching with Naomi 1:00 Discussion Groups 2:00 Bingo Time 3:00 Snacks and say goodbye	**5 Birthday of Traffic Lights** 9:00 Coffee Klatch & Puzzles 9:30 News & Discussion 10:00 Match Game 10:00 Creative Corner with Lynda 11:00 Aerobic Dancing 1:00 Tiny Nook Tea Room Event 2:00 Joking Around 3:00 Snacks and say goodbye	**6 Lucille Ball's Birthday** 9:00 Coffee Klatch & Puzzles 9:30 News & Discussion 10:00 Yoga with Craige 10:00 Art Class 11:00 Work out Video 1:00 Chuck Stevenson 3:00 Snacks and say goodbye	**7 National Lighthouse Day** 9:00 Coffee Klatch & Puzzles 9:30 News & Discussion 10:00 Knit & Chat with Anna 10:00 Shirley Hedrick 11:00 Aerobic Dancing 1:00 Connie Molino at the Piano 2:00 Circle of Friends 3:00 Snacks and say goodbye	**8 8-08-08 Lucky Day** 9:00 Coffee Klatch & Puzzles 9:30 News & Discussion 10:00 Anna's Sewing Bee 10:00 Bob's Band 11:00 Easy Exercise with Stephanie 1:00 David Kramer Music 2:00 Bingo Time 3:00 Snacks and say goodbye
11 9:00 Coffee Klatch & Puzzles 9:30 News & Discussion 10:00 Yoga with Phyllis 10:00 Crafts Club with Anna 11:00 Word Game with Naomi 1:00 Rick Herrera Floral Design 2:00 Bingo Time 3:00 Snacks and say goodbye	**12 Vinyl Record Day** 9:00 Coffee Klatch & Puzzles 9:30 News & Discussion 10:00 Price is Right 10:30 Chuck Stevenson 11:00 Aerobic Dancing 1:00 Dancing to the Oldies 2:00 Joking Around 3:00 Snacks and say goodbye	**13 Int'l Left Hander's Day** 9:00 Coffee Klatch & Puzzles 9:30 News & Discussion 10:00 Charades, Discussion Group 10:00 Art Class 11:00 Work out Video 1:00 Olympics Celebration 2:00 Bingo Time 3:00 Snacks and say goodbye	**14** 9:00 Coffee Klatch & Puzzles 9:30 News & Discussion 10:00 Knit & Chat with Anna 10:00 Lee Nemeroff Tibet & China 11:00 Aerobic Dancing 1:00 David Kramer 2:00 Circle of Friends 3:00 Snacks and say goodbye	**15 National Relaxation Day** 9:00 Coffee Klatch & Puzzles 9:30 News & Discussion 10:00 Anna's Sewing Bee 10:00 Bob's Band 11:00 Easy Exercise with Stephanie 1:00 Liam O'Brien 2:00 Bingo Time 3:00 Snacks and say goodbye
18 9:00 Coffee Klatch & Puzzles 9:30 News & Discussion 10:00 Yoga with Ruth 10:00 Crafts Club with Anna 11:00 Word Game with Naomi 1:00 Fritz – Keychains 2:00 Bingo Time 3:00 Snacks and say goodbye	**19 Potato Day** 9:00 Coffee Klatch & Puzzles 9:30 News & Discussion 10:00 Love on a Leash/Christian Life 10:00 Crossword Puzzle 11:00 Aerobic Dancing 1:00 John & Rebecca Broadway Tunes 2:00 Circle of Friends 3:00 Snacks and say goodbye	**20 Lemonade's Birthday** 9:00 Coffee Klatch & Puzzles 9:30 News & Discussion 10:00 Art Class 10:00 Connie's Doll Collection 11:00 Work out Video 1:00 Chuck Stevenson Big Band 2:00 Bingo Time 3:00 Snacks and say goodbye	**21 Poet Day** 9:00 Coffee Klatch & Puzzles 9:30 News & Discussion 10:00 Knit & Chat with Anna 10:00 4 H Club 11:00 Aerobic Dancing 1:00 Marty Albert Songs 2:00 Circle of Friends 3:00 Snacks and say goodbye	**22 Be an Angel Day** 9:00 Coffee Klatch & Puzzles 9:30 News & Discussion 10:00 Anna's Sewing Bee 10:00 Bob's Band 11:00 Easy Exercise with Stephanie 1:00 Shakespeare 2:00 Bingo Time 3:00 Snacks and say goodbye
25 Kiss and Make Up Day 9:00 Coffee Klatch 9:30 News & Discussion 10:00 Yoga with Ilene 10:00 Crafts Club with Anna 11:00 Word Game with Naomi 1:00 Bill Carter Songs 2:00 Bingo Time 3:00 Snacks and say goodbye	**26 Women's Equality Day** 9:00 Coffee Klatch & Puzzles 9:30 News & Discussion 10:00 Creative Corner with Lynda 10:30 Chuck Stevenson 11:00 Aerobic Dancing 1:00 David Kramer 2:00 Joking Around 3:00 Snacks and say goodbye	**27** 9:00 Coffee Klatch 9:30 News & Discussion 10:00 Art Class 10:00 Katie Cook at the Piano 11:00 Work out Video 1:00 Fred La Porte Sings 2:00 Bingo Time 3:00 Snacks and say goodbye	**28** 9:00 Coffee Klatch 9:30 News & Discussion 10:00 Knit & Chat with Anna 10:00 Wislock Family Slings 11:00 Aerobic Dancing 1:00 Ralph Cola 2:00 Circle of Friends 3:00 Snacks and say goodbye	**29 More Herbs, Less Salt Day** 9:00 Coffee Klatch 9:30 News & Discussion 10:00 Anna's Sewing Bee 10:00 Bob's Band 11:00 Easy Exercise with Stephanie 1:00 Trish & Nancy Songs 2:00 Bingo Time 3:00 Snacks and say goodbye

Figure 21: Senior Concerns Monthly Calendar

Stage 5: Moderately Severe Cognitive Decline/Early-Stage Alzheimer's

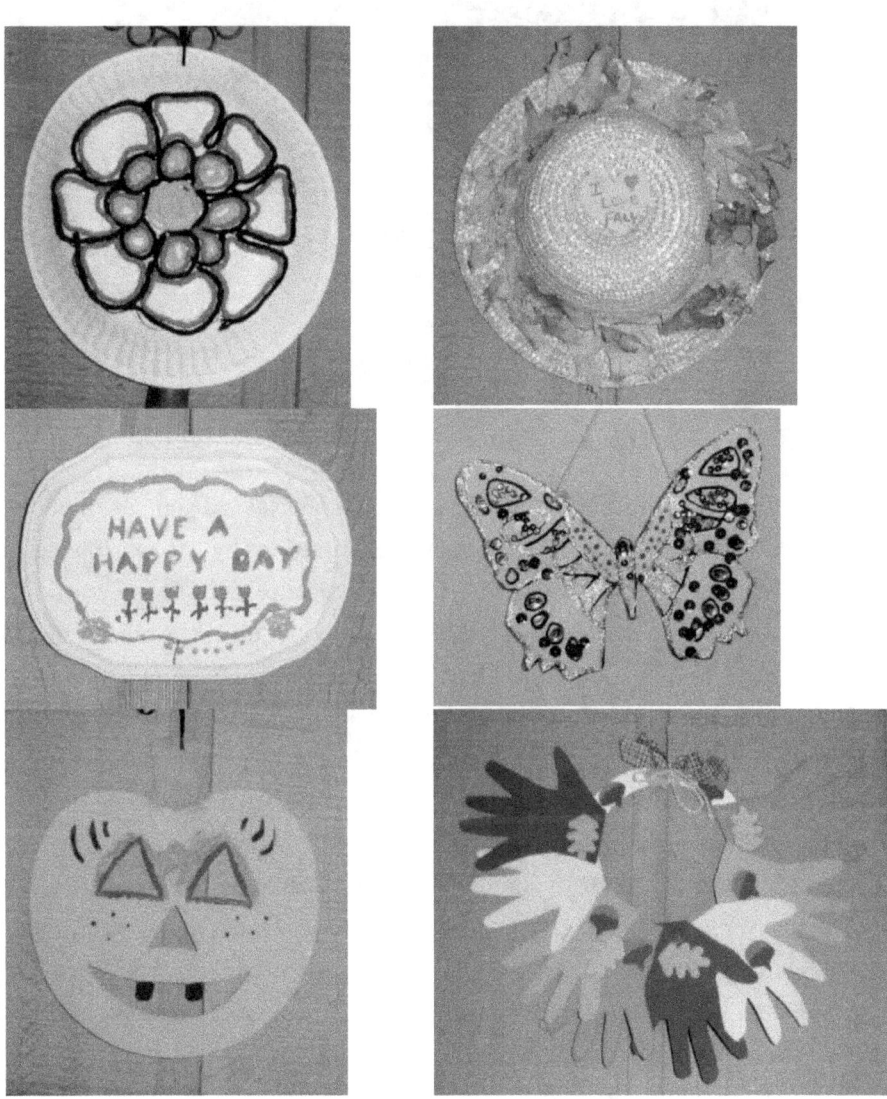

Figure 22: Creative Art Olive Made at Senior Concerns

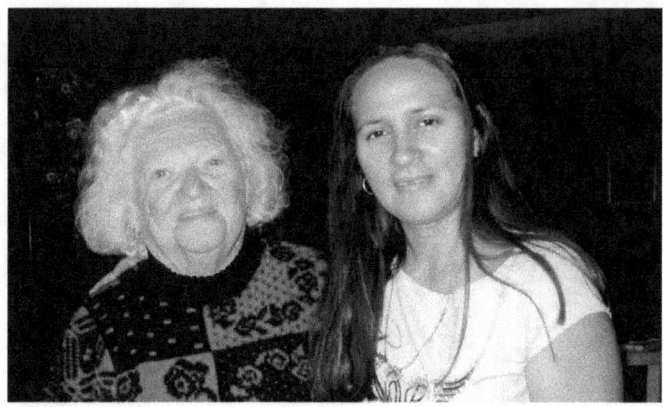

Figure 23: Olive & Primary In-Home Caregiver, Ana

During the day, Mother frequently visited with Bea Madison, a neighbor who was also diagnosed with Alzheimer's and cared for by her son John and Claribel, a live-in caregiver. Claribel, who is a registered nurse in Peru and Spain, was also studying to obtain an RN License in the U.S. At this time, Olive helped Claribel with her English. Claribel passed the "English as a Second Language (ESL) Test" as part of her requirements to obtain her registered nursing (RN) license in California. Later, Claribel passed and received her California RN License, became a U.S. citizen and now owns her own private board and care home.

During April/May 2002, a neighbor at the lake attempted to take advantage of mother by requesting a zoning change. The request was turned down by the zoning board because of letters sent by myself and the other adjoining neighbor. The process took me about six weeks to resolve. This was the third attempt I observed of a person trying to take advantage of an elderly woman with failing health.

Stage 5: Moderately Severe Cognitive Decline/Early-Stage Alzheimer's

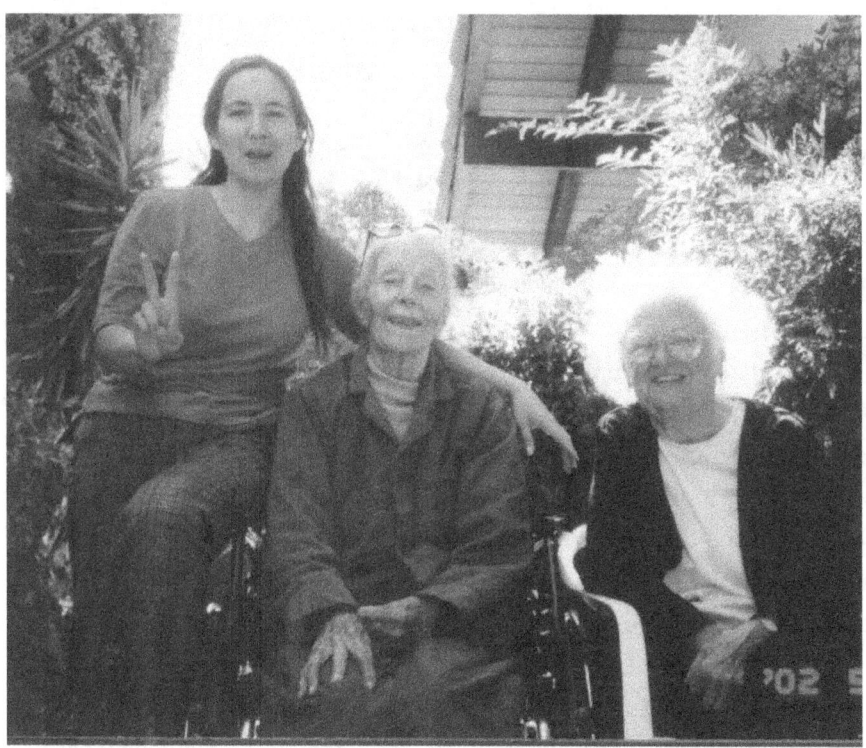

Figure 24: Neighbors, Claribel, Bea and Olive, May 11, 2002

During June 2002, I helped move my daughter Shelby and her belongings to Oregon and then a year later back to Westlake. Mother stayed with my ex-wife Nina during the return trip. While I was gone, Mother experienced a mild stroke on June 27, 2002. After the stroke, the double vision returned. During July mother was examined by a Neuro-Opthalmologist at the USC Medical Center. The Neuro-Ophthalmologist's conclusion was that mother's stroke had affected her number three optic nerve. That was why she was seeing multiple images. The doctor stated further, "In approximately ninety days Olive's vision will return to normal." Exactly as the doctor predicted, Olive's sight returned to normal after ninety days.

During June 2002, we placed the lake property up for sale. Mother did not have a problem walking at this time except she constantly looked down at the sidewalk and rarely looked at the view or surroundings.

In August of 2002 we returned to Wisconsin to attend the funeral of the man with whom mother had had a ten year relationship. Each of their spouses had died suddenly and unexpectedly. Olive and Bob, who were neighbors, enjoyed each other's companionship before he met and married another woman. It was a good relationship for Olive and Bob. Additionally, we took care of some personal business. Afterward we went to the County Fair and I pushed mother around the grounds in a wheel chair. At the fair mother visited with several relatives and friends.

During this trip to Wisconsin, Olive continued to walk by herself, an exercise she thoroughly enjoyed. On three occasions, she wondered off, got lost or lost track of time. Each time a friend either drove her home or called me to come and take her home. Additionally, two mornings I woke up and found her sitting naked; the first time in a recliner in the living room and the second time, before sunrise, in a chair in the backyard. Another morning before sunrise, I found mother asleep on the bathroom floor. She had apparently woke up during the night to go to the bathroom and slipped and fell or just forgot where she was and laid down on the floor and went back to sleep. Many times I asked mother to not constantly go up to the attic or down to the basement for fear that she might fall but she continued because she could no longer remember our conversations or follow directions. One morning she fell while walking out of the garage to hang clothes on the line. I took her to the local hospital where they took an x-ray of her arm. Luckily, no bones were broken. The doctor ended up placing a splint on Olive's wrist to protect the sprain and help it heal.

During October 2002, we sold the lake property. Cousin Don helped me move the furniture and personal belongings from the lake to my mother's home in Elkhorn. As a result, I gave the red runabout boat that my parents bought before I returned from Vietnam, to my cousin Don's son, Tim. This was the first of many sad days. As I stood on top of the boathouse watching the boat disappearing down the lake, I realized that one of my long term dreams had just vanished. I had always planned to divide my retirement time

Stage 5: Moderately Severe Cognitive Decline/Early-Stage Alzheimer's

between this beautiful lakeside cottage and my home in Westlake Village. I cried that day. Later, my mother and I drove down to a launch where my cousin was planning to take the boat out of the lake and place it on a trailer for transportation to Tim's home. Near the boat launch I got out of the car but left the engine and heater running since it was cold outside. I asked mother to remain in the car while I helped Don and Tim. Instead, a few minutes later, Olive opened the door and wandered off. As a result, I ended up searching for Olive for a half an hour until I found her. We then drove home. Selling the cottage was a difficult emotional experience for both my mother and me. However, several days later mother seemed to forget the sale and was back to normal happy, optimistic self as you can see in Figure 25: Lifelong Friend Kirt & Olive, October 28, 2002 on page 93.

During October, Olive's Sister Betty and her daughter Karen came to visit and brought a bouquet of colorful fragrant flowers for mother. Olive was very excited by the beautiful flowers. Later Olive pointed to some dolls and said to her sister, "Do you remember these dolls on the couch." Betty said, "No." Olive continued, "Well, they used to be ours when we were young." Later Aunt Betty told me that the dolls came from one of their mother's spending sprees and that they had been stored in their mother's basement for fifteen years." At the end of the visit, Karen said to me, "Bob, your mother seems unusually anxious."

In early November we left for California. It was very difficult for mother to leave the house that she and my dad had built from scratch. Additionally, we had sold the lake property. I think mother was capable of realizing that this might be the last time she would be able to enjoy her home or lake property. Before we departed for California, cousins Howard and Betty and Don and June met with Olive to discuss her need to go with me to California since she was not capable of caring for herself any longer. Both couples had been through this experience with their parents. Additionally, the morning of the trip to the airport, my lifelong friend Kirt took Olive for a walk and encouraged her to go to California. We ate lunch at Midway Airport in Chicago. Afterwards, Olive had to use the bathroom. Upon walking out of the bathroom, Olive walked past me without me noticing her. She became lost and wandered around the airport for three hours. Finally, security paged me and I was able to locate her. After rescheduling the flight five or six times, we finally left for California in November 2002.

August 2003, I held a party at my home in Westlake to celebrate mother's birthday. Approximately twenty five people attended the party, including my ex-wife, my two daughters, friends and neighbors. Mother thoroughly enjoyed the celebration.

From August 2003 through August 2004, Olive attended Senior Concerns, a day care center for dementia patients in Thousand Oaks, California. On Friday nights Olive loved to go to the Westlake Promenade and listen to live bands. If Senior Concerns staff members attended, they would often ask mother to dance. Early in 2003, a live-in caregiver moved into my home to help with mother's care. Mother started to walk with the aid of a cane in 2002. During 2003 Olive depended on the cane all the time.

May 2003 I flew to Wisconsin and drove mother's 1993 Buick Skylark with less than 20,000 miles back to California. During this time, a caregiver looked after mother. The Saturday of Memorial Day weekend 2003, my daughter, Aubrey, Mother and I ate breakfast at the International House of Pancakes. With a caregiver taking care of my mother, my daughter Aubrey and I could spend Saturday night camping at Joshua Tree National Park. Mother was fine during our absence eating food I prepared before we left for our one-day trip.

During the late summer of 2003 while my friend Ken was visiting, Olive came out of the bathroom with the waistband of her underpants over her head and her arms sticking out of one of the leg openings. A couple of weeks later while Shelby was visiting with a new boyfriend, mother came out of the bathroom with nothing on except a bra. Mother, seemingly realizing something was wrong, turned around and returned to the bathroom where I helped her get dressed and we walked back together to the living room.

Stage 5: Moderately Severe Cognitive Decline/Early-Stage Alzheimer's

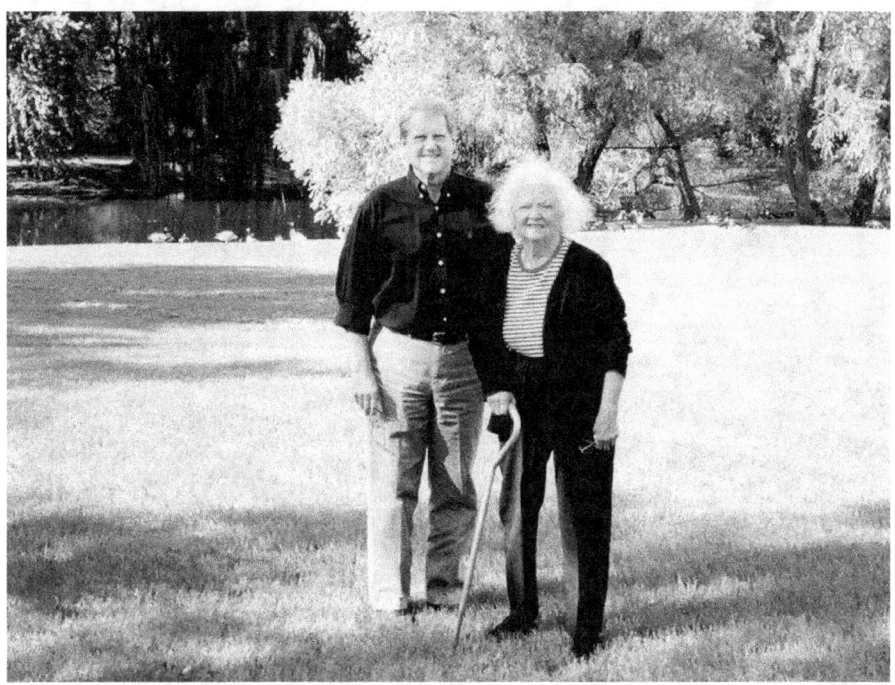

Figure 25: Lifelong Friend Kirt & Olive, October 28, 2002

Typically, Olive would go to bed between nine and ten o'clock and rise between six-thirty and seven-thirty. Beginning in the fall of 2003 mother began crying occasionally at night before she would go to sleep. When this would happen, I would cuddle her in my arms and ask, "Why are you crying mother?" There would be no response. "What is making you cry?" Still no answer from mother, so I would then kiss her and tuck her into bed. This must have been an absolutely terrifying time for mother to realize her mental capacity was rapidly declining. This was also a confusing time for me as a caregiver because I felt so helpless since there was nothing I could do to make the situation better or go away.

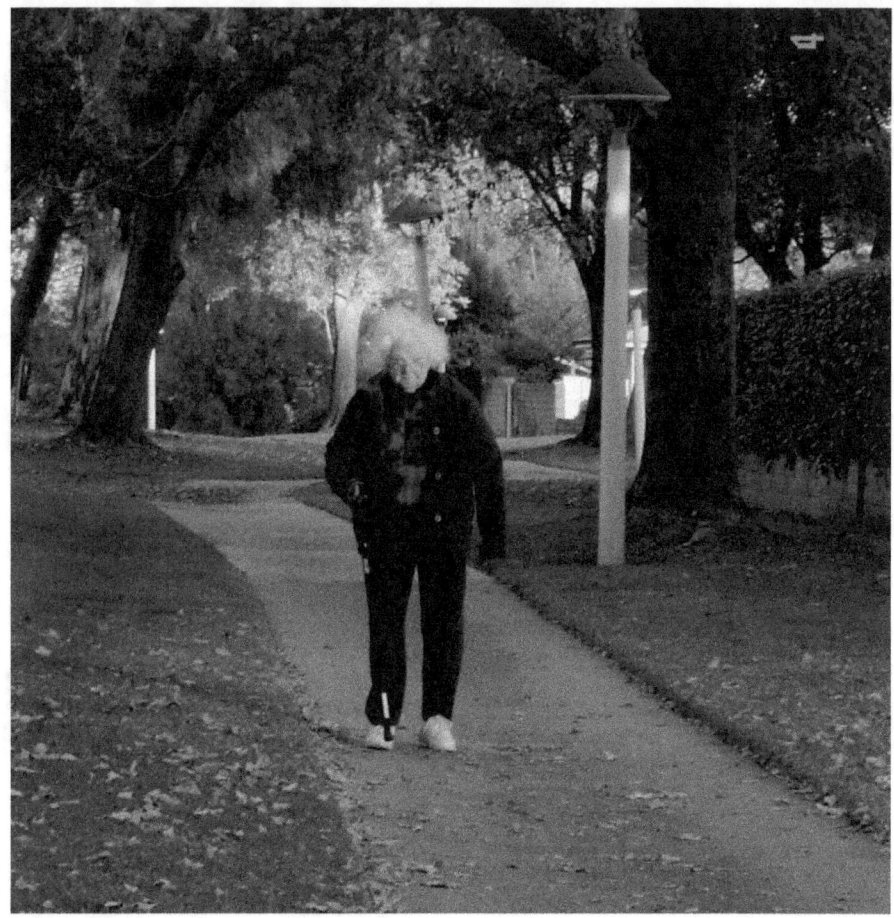

Figure 26: Olive Walking next to Bob's Home, December 4, 2003

I believe you can see in Figure 26 above, the growing expression of frustration on Olive's face as the result of Alzheimer disease. Figure 27 on page 95 is a picture of Olive resting in Bennett Park during one of her many walks. However, there were many joyous occasions during this stage when mother was very happy and seemed very normal as you can see in Figure 28 and Figure 29, on page 96 and Figure 30 and Figure 31 on page 97.

Stage 5: Moderately Severe Cognitive Decline/Early-Stage Alzheimer's

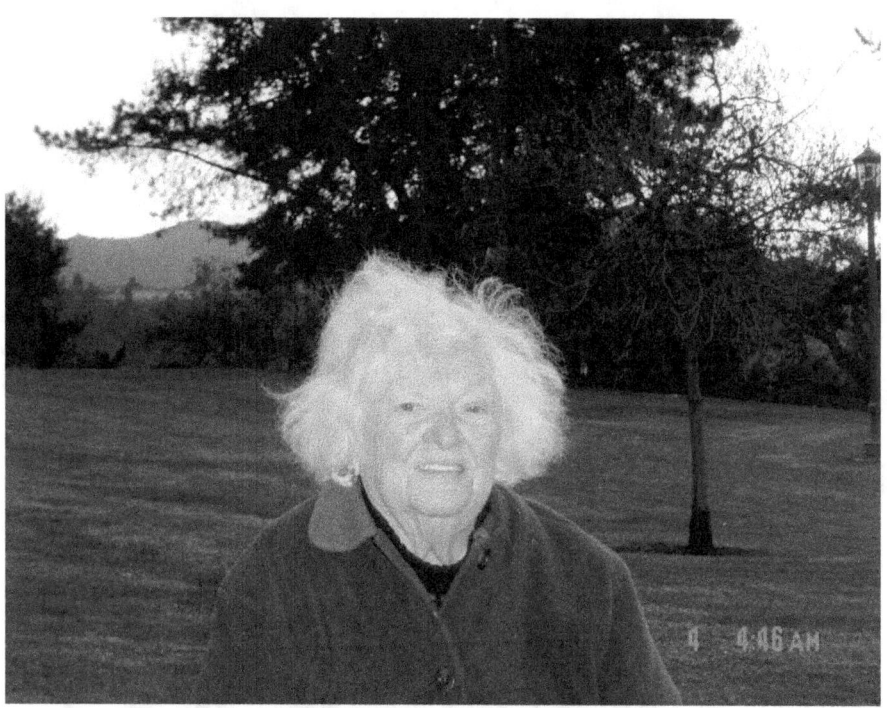

Figure 27: Olive Resting at Bennett Park, Westlake Village, CA, December 4, 2003

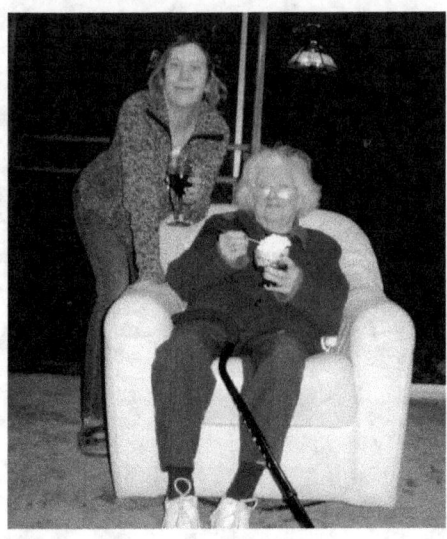

Figure 28: Youngest Granddaughter Shelby & Olive, December 11, 2003

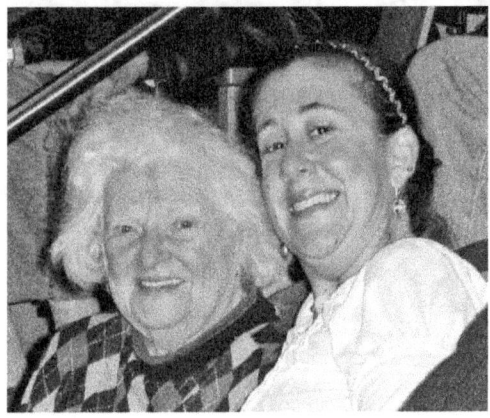

Figure 29: Olive & Oldest Grandaughter Aubrey at Willie Nelson Concert, Thousand Oaks Performing Arts Center, 11/30/2003

Stage 5: Moderately Severe Cognitive Decline/Early-Stage Alzheimer's

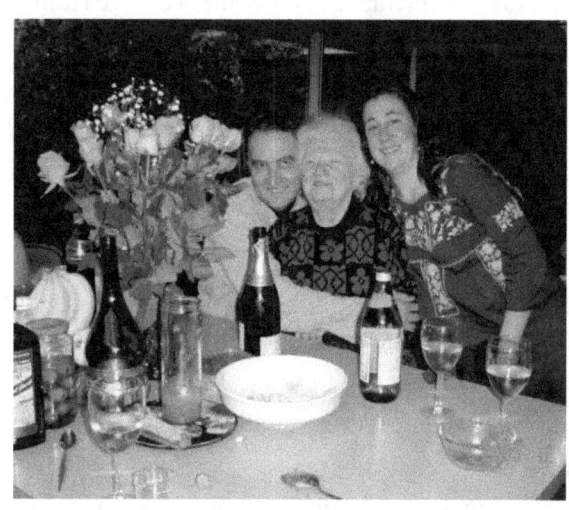

Figure 30: Friend, Ken Bayus, Olive & Aubrey, December 31, 2003

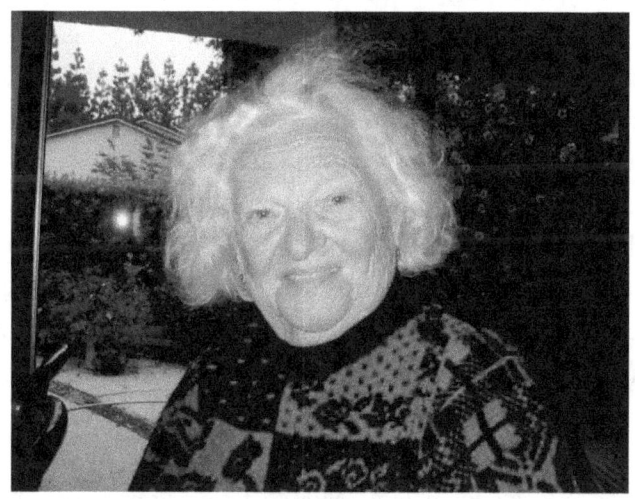

Figure 31: Olive at Bob's Home, Westlake Village, CA, March 6, 2004

Alzheimer's--What My Mother's Caregiving Taught Me

One evening during September 2004 while we were sitting in the family room, mother asked me, "What is your relationship to me?" This surprised me and was the first sign to me that sometimes mother no longer realized that I was her son. A week later, I made a comment to mother about the beauty of the paintings on the family room wall. Mother was a skilled artist and had painted the pictures to give to me as Christmas and birthday gifts. I had the paintings displayed in the family room along with other paintings she had done that we had moved from her home in Wisconsin. I said to mother, "I notice you enjoy looking at the paintings. Did you ever have an opportunity to meet the artist?" Mother replied, "No." This indicated to me that mother's memory was deteriorating rapidly. At this point, she was not even aware she painted these beautiful scenes.

Early in 2004, mother was requiring more and more assistance with daily living. Also, during early 2004, Olive became lost for the first time since she had been living with me. She walked into a neighbor's house similar to mine but a block away where the couple was watching the evening news. Knowing the situation, the couple said, "Olive, how nice it is for you to stop by and visit us. Would you like some tea?" Mother responded, "That would be very nice." The husband then slipped into the study, phoned me and said, "I bet you are looking for your mother." I said, "How do you know?" I then walked over to the neighbor's home and joined them for tea. Afterward, mother and I walked home. One day during the summer mother went for her daily walk and became lost a second time. A neighbor across the greenbelt phoned to tell me where my mother was. He had obtained the number to call from the information provided on the "Safe Return Bracelet" that mother always wore on her right wrist. Safe Return is a vital program in which to enroll a person suffering from dementia. If a loved one gets lost, the program helps to locate them 24/7. More details on this program can be found starting on page 124. Shortly after the second incident, Olive stopped walking alone and would sit in front of the house during the afternoon and talk to neighbors and school children as they passed the house after classes. Another elderly man who rode a bicycle would often ride by, stop and talk to

Stage 5: Moderately Severe Cognitive Decline/Early-Stage Alzheimer's

mother. It was very thoughtful on his part and mother enjoyed their visits.

During April 2004, I returned to Wisconsin to check on Olive's home. While I was away, the caregiver woke Olive up one morning to go to Senior Concerns. She bathed, dressed and prepared breakfast for Olive. Because the caregiver had to leave, she left my mother sitting in front of the house waiting for transportation to Senior Concerns. Mother, instead of waiting for the transport, went back in the house, used the bathroom and then had lain down on her bed and fell asleep. When the driver pulled up to the house to pick up Olive and she was not waiting, he got out of his vehicle and walked up to the house. There, he found the front door ajar so he walked in and found Olive, dressed for Senior Concerns, asleep in bed. The driver then woke up Olive and drove her to Senior Concerns. That evening while my daughter Shelby was visiting for dinner with her grandmother, the sheriff and a deputy showed up because someone had called family protective services. The two police officers then proceeded without probable cause or a search warrant to inspect the entire house by looking under beds, in closets, the pantry, refrigerator and freezer. When I learned of the situation from my daughter, I returned home and spent a frustrating couple of weeks attempting to resolve the situation. The officers never gave me the courtesy of a phone call or provided me with documentation on their search which I still consider an invasion of privacy.

During the summer and fall of 2004, mother continued to decline. I would turn on the television to watch the news and would notice mother looking out the window or at the walls or floor. She would pick up a newspaper but was unable to mentally process the contents. She also had difficulty holding the newspaper. Olive continually thought she had to go to the bathroom. During August, Senior Concerns called and asked me to come in for a conference. During the meeting, the director said, "Olive is requiring more support than we are capable of offering and we will no longer be able to offer her day care services. Olive now requires constant one-on-one care that Senior Concerns is not staffed to handle." Similarly, the live-in caregiver said it was more than she could handle and moved out the same month. Olive's memory difficulties continued to decline and significant personality changes emerged requiring a need for more extensive help with customary daily activities.

During August, mother developed constipation problems. One Friday during that month, her constipation problem became so severe that I had to take mother to the local emergency ward. We spent seven hours there to get the problem resolved. During the treatments, mother was in a lot of pain and even called the doctor a "son of a bitch" when he was not present. A comment of this type was something I had never heard from mother in the past. While still in the emergency room she said, "If I ever get out of this God damn place, I am going straight back to Wisconsin." After this emergency experience, I included senna and psyllium capsules that I purchased from a health foods store, along with her other prescription medications from a pharmacy to insure Olive's regular bowl movements. Senna is a natural laxative. Psyllium is mainly used as a dietary fiber, which is not absorbed by the small intestine. The purely mechanical action of psyllium mucilage absorbs excess water while stimulating normal bowel elimination as a constipation remedy.

September 2004, while my friend Ken was visiting, Olive developed diarrhea, which ended up all over the bed, carpet and bathroom. When I awoke at three in the morning, mother was finger painting on the bathroom wall with her feces. I cleaned everything, gave Olive a shower, dressed her in a clean nightgown, changed the bedding, did laundry three times that day and cut the carpet out of the bathroom. That evening I went to dinner with my friend Ken while a caregiver looked after mother. At dinner, Ken said, "I don't know how you deal with this situation. I couldn't handle the stress of caring for anyone."

I tried to handle the situation by myself during late August, September and October but realized it was more than I was capable of handling.

During Stage 5, mother showed all the behaviors listed at the beginning of this section.

Stage 5: Moderately Severe Cognitive Decline/Early-Stage Alzheimer's

Placement

Shortly thereafter my friend Roger, from the local Alzheimer support group, joined me to check out board and care facilities for our mothers. We settled on a board and care facility for my mother that was spotlessly clean, had responsible caregivers and prepared and served delicious fresh food. Before the admission, I even went to the extent of checking out the refrigerator and found it was stocked with fresh fruit and vegetables. I felt at this Board and Care, Olive would be safe, clean and her nutritional needs would be met.

On Wednesday, November 10, 2004, after researching and visiting board and care homes and after much deliberation, I place mother at Leisure Living (LLB&C) in Agoura Hills, California. Immediately I felt a sense of relief and then guilt from placing my mother. However, it was the correct action to take at the time for the wellbeing of both of us.

My decision to place mother in an independent board and care facility was based on the following:

- The behavioral changes accompanying Alzheimer's were causing daily chaos and becoming difficult to handle.
- My energy was beginning to run low nearly every day. At the time, I did not realize that some of the fatigue was coming from undiagnosed cancer.
- I was exhausted nearly all the time. I also realized that when I was continually tired, I was not capable of making the best decisions.
- I felt a professional staff of full time caregivers could provide better quality care for Olive's day-to-day needs (cleanliness, exercise, nutrition and safety).
- Placement would allow me to focus on managing Olive's overall health care.

The following is the background leading up to my Uncle Ray's placement decision by his daughter and her husband. First, Uncle Ray began repetitively asking his daughter Betty, who was also his caregiver, "Who is the person in the bathroom window who keeps watching me shave everyday." Unbeknown to Uncle Ray it was his own reflection in the mirror.

Earlier while Uncle Ray was still living alone, he would forget to turn off the gas on the kitchen range after he finished cooking. Often, you could smell gas as you entered his home. Neighbors got concerned because Uncle Ray enjoyed trap shooting as a hobby and he reloaded his own ammunition in the basement. Neighbors thought that one day he was going to blow-up the entire neighborhood; either from leaving the gas for his kitchen stove on or from the explosives in his basement. They complained to Betty and her husband. First, they sold Uncle Ray's home and moved Uncle Ray to an apartment. However, the problems continued and then he started to think that his wife, who had been dead for ten years, was visiting him. Next, his daughter had Uncle Ray move in with them. This went well for a while until one morning when Howard, Betty's husband, woke up in the morning and bathed Uncle Ray as usual. After Uncle Ray was bathed and dressed, Howard took a shower. When Howard finished showering, he came out of the bathroom and saw Uncle Ray, who was mad at Betty, coming out of the kitchen with a frying pan in his hand. After the incident, Howard talked to Betty and they agreed for the need to place Uncle Ray. That week they admitted Uncle Ray to a local skilled nursing facility where he lived until he passed away.

My cousin Elmer at age eighty he began to have memory problems. In early 2003 Elmer told me that a man stopped at his house and knocked at his door. Allegedly, the man asked Elmer if he was interested in helping him milk cows for some extra money. Elmer said, "Sure." According to Elmer, initially the man picked him up at his house around three o'clock in the afternoon. This went well for a while. Then according to Elmer, he started coming later and later. On one night when he arrived at eleven o'clock, Elmer answered the door and said he told him, "Go to hell, I'm not milking any cows." Then, according to Elmer, the man knocked down the door and beat Elmer up. Elmer then called 911. When I arrived back in California, I was not sure how to break this news to his son Larry. Finally, I called Larry who was spending the winter in Arizona. I told Larry that I stopped by and visited his dad and then told him about the incident with his father. Larry said, "I believe you, since the police called me and said that dad had called five or six times. However, when the police arrived, Elmer was lying on the floor unharmed and they could not detect any sign of break-in or a scuffle." Larry then proceeded to tell me that he had spoken to Elmer and he said that, "strange people were in his back yard." Larry asked, "What is strange about them?" Elmer replied, "They don't have any bodies, just unusual heads." Larry returned home a few days later and upon arrival at Elmer's home, Larry and his wife sat down on the couch with Elmer between them. Elmer then said, "You will probably think that I am crazy but Violet, my wife, is sitting across from us." Larry and Lana looked at each other confused because no one was sitting across from them. However, Elmer believed that Violet was sitting in the room with them. Maybe her spirit was there trying to protect him—we know so little about the paranormal. Later a caregiver was hired and Elmer was placed on medication. Because the caregiver did not work out and because of Elmer's declining mental state, he moved to a nursing home and his home was sold. The delusions have since gone away with the aid of medications. However, Elmer continues to live in the nursing home because he requires assistance with his daily needs.

For each person the time and criteria of placement in either a board and care or a skilled nursing facility or private nursing home will vary. The key is to know yourself, your limits and set your own criteria for placement and be comfortable with your decision in the long term.

Stage 5: Recommendation for Caregivers
Extremely High Priority on Quality Time Together

This stage will be your final opportunity for quality two-way communication with your loved one. There will be times when communications will be perfectly normal. However, there will also be times when the person may drift away and not be present for the conversation. Be patient, non-verbal communication begins to be important at this stage. Things as simple as smiling at each other, touch, frequent hugs or rubbing their hands, head, shoulders or feet; stimulation of smell by flowers or food preparation; sound stimulation by playing familiar music, humming or singing tunes from their past when they were in their twenties to fifties are all effective.

Caregiver Health

It is very important in this stage to be working on a program to build physical and mental endurance. A person is not aware of it but the physical and mental stress from caregiving will wear you down. Respites, or brief night or weekend periods of rest and recovery away from caregiving are extremely important.

Respite

A respite may be as simple of having a friend spend an evening with your loved one while you go out to dinner or see a movie by yourself or with friends. Alternatively, it may mean placing the loved one overnight or a weekend at a care facility. These periods for the loved one at a care facility are a good way for accessing and transitioning to a care facility when the time comes.

Diagnosis

Diagnosis as discussed in the previous section is the most important activity to be completed in stage four. If it was not done in stage 4, now is the time to schedule a full neuropsychological diagnosis (see Appendix C: Diagnosing Alzheimer's, on page 239). Equally important, is the medical institution you choose and the qualifications and experience of the doctors who perform the testing. My personal recommendation is to have the assessment performed at one of the hospitals listed in Appendix D: Alzheimer Disease Research Centers, on page 259. At one of these Centers a quality assessment can be accurately performed. Many local hospitals do not have the equipment, supporting personnel or day-to-day expertise to routinely performing this assessment.

Once the diagnosis is complete, you are able to make plans and arrangements for the future. It is important to have these plans in place

Stage 5: Moderately Severe Cognitive Decline/Early-Stage Alzheimer's

ideally during stage four or at the latest, stage five. Otherwise, you will become completely overwhelmed by the caregiving demands of Alzheimer's disease.

Decision to Change Living Arrangement

The decision to change one's living arrangement is difficult, especially if the love one has resided in their home for a long period. It is even more difficult when moving away to another city or state. However, this is another one of the many difficult decisions a caregiver and the loved one must face. It is of primary importance for the person afflicted with Alzheimer's disease to be near a loved one who can oversee their care.

Medications

A note to all caregivers that one of the best sources of information on various drugs is MedlinePlus, A Service of The National Library of Medicine and The National Institutes of Health.[51]

Treatment to Insure Bowel Regularity

Psyllium

Psyllium is mainly used as a dietary fiber, which is not absorbed by the small intestine. The purely mechanical action of psyllium mucilage absorbs excess water while stimulating normal bowel elimination. Although its main use has been as a laxative, it is more appropriately termed a true dietary fiber.

Senna

Senna acts as a purgative and is similar to aloe and rhubarb in having as active ingredients anthraquinone derivatives and their glucosides. The latter are called sennosides or senna glycosides. Senna acts on the lower bowel, and is especially useful in alleviating constipation. It increases the peristaltic movements of the colon.

---

[51] Source: National Institute of Aging, U.S. National Institute of Health, at Internet address: http://medlineplus.gov/.

Alzheimer's Medication

- Aricept®)
- Exelon®)
- Razadyne®
- Namenda®
- Cognex®

No treatment has been proven to stop AD. However, for some people in the early and middle stages of the disease, the drugs donepezil (Aricept®), rivastigmine (Exelon®), or galantamine (Razadyne®, formerly known as Reminyl®) may help prevent some symptoms from becoming worse for a limited time in some patients. Another drug, tacrine (Cognex®) was approved by the Food and Drug Administration (FDA), but it is no longer actively marketed by the manufacturer. In addition, the drug, memantine (Namenda®), has been approved to treat moderate to severe AD. Namenda is also limited in its effects. In addition, the FDA recently approved the use of donepezil to treat moderate to severe AD.

In addition, some medicines may help control behavioral symptoms related to AD such as bowl regularity, sleeplessness, agitation, wandering, anxiety, depression and pain. Treating these symptoms often makes patients more comfortable and makes their care easier for caregivers.

Alternative Alzheimer's Herbs

Curcumin

Curcumin inhibits formation of amyloid beta oligomers and fibrils, binds plaques, and reduces amyloid in test tube studies. Researchers at UCLA found that Curcumin taken for Alzheimer's diseases might reduce oridation damage and inflammation, reduce amyloid accumulation and synaptic marker loss.[52]

Currently, the National Institute on Health is conducting a pilot clinical

---

[52] Curcumin & Alzheimer's and Cancer, ongoing studies at Alzheimer's research lab, UCLA, plus human drug trial.

Stage 5: Moderately Severe Cognitive Decline/Early-Stage Alzheimer's

trial to evaluate curcumin at UCLA.

Huperzine-A

Huperzine-A, is a naturally occurring sesquiterpene alkaloid found in the extracts of the firmoss Huperzia serrata. The botanical has been used in China for centuries for the treatment of swelling, fever and blood disorders. Recently in clinical trials in China, it has demonstrated neuroprotective effects. It is currently being investigated as a possible treatment for diseases characterized by neurodegeneration – particularly Alzheimer's disease.

Huperzine-A has attracted the attention of Western medical science. It has been found to be an inhibitor of the enzyme acetylcholinesterase. This is the same mechanism of action of pharmaceutical drugs such as galantamine and donepezil used to treat Alzheimer's disease.

Clinical trials in China have shown that Huperzine-A is comparably effective to the drugs currently on the market, and may even be a bit safer in terms of side effects. Currently, the National Institute on Aging is conducting a Phase II clinical trial to evaluate the safety and efficiency of Huperzine-A in the treatment of Alzheimer's disease in a randomized controlled trial of its effect on cognitive function. One study is currently being conducted at the University of Southern California (USC).

Ginkgo Biloba

Among alternative therapies, Ginkgo Biloba, a tree long valued in China for its medicinal properties, has shown some promise. Several European studies suggest that ginkgo may offer both cognitive and behavioral benefits, including alleviation of anxiety.

Antidepressant Medications

- Prozac
- Paxil
- Celexa
- Pamelor
- Zoloft

Antidepressants, such as Prozac, Paxil, Celexa, Pamelor and Zoloft, are used to treat depression. Side effects of these medicines can include drowsiness, dry mouth, constipation, and anxiety.

Anti-Anxiety Medications

- Ativan
- BuSpar
- Serax
- Xanax

These medications, which include Ativan, BuSpar, Serax, and Xanax, often cause drowsiness.

Antipsychotics Medication

Use in Older Adults[53]

Studies have shown that older adults with dementia (a brain disorder that affects the ability to remember, think clearly, communicate and perform daily activities and may also cause changes in mood and personality) who take antipsychotics (medications for mental illness) such as quetiapine have an increased risk of death during treatment. If you experience any of the following symptoms: slow or difficult speech, sudden dizziness or faintness, weakness or numbness of an arm or leg, call your doctor immediately.

Antipsychotics Medication are known among Caregivers as "Caregiver Bust," because their cost exceeds $150/month. The medications are frequently prescribed to keep patients quiet and manageable.

Quetiapine is not approved by the Food and Drug Administration (FDA) for the treatment of behavioral problems in older adults with dementia. Talk to the doctor who prescribed this medication if you, a family member, or someone you care for has dementia and is taking quetiapine. For more information, visit the FDA website: http://www.fda.gov/cder

- Haloperidol (Haldol),
- Risperdal

---

[53] MedlinePlus, A Service of The National Library of Medicine and The National Institutes of Health, September 2008.

Stage 5: Moderately Severe Cognitive Decline/Early-Stage Alzheimer's

- Zyprexa
- Clozaril
- Geodon
- Seroquel

Antipsychotics medicines used to treat paranoia and confusion are called neuroleptics or antipsychotics. Examples of these medicines are haloperidol (Haldol), Risperdal, Zyprexa, Clozaril, Geodon and Seroquel. Side effects can include drowsiness, rigidity, and unusual movements.

Insomnia (Sleep Disorder) Medications

- Ambien
- Diphenhydramine, Brand Name(s): Benadryl, Genahist, Sominex, Unisom
- Halcion
- Lunesta
- Restoril
- Rozerem
- Sonata

Extreme Pain Medications

The following medications are used to relieve moderate to severe pain:

- Oxycodin
- Morphine

DRUG	MAY NOT BE SAFE FOR ALZHEIMER PATIENT IF THEY:	CONSIDERATIONS
Eszopiclone (Lunesta)	Have a history of drug or alcohol abuse, depression, lung disease, or a condition that affects metabolism.	May be used for a longer period of time than zolpidem or zaleplon. High-fat meals may slow absorption of the drug and make it less effective. Stopping the drug abruptly may cause withdrawal symptoms such as anxiety, unusual dreams, stomach and muscle cramps, nausea, vomiting, sweating, and shakiness.
Ramelteon (Rozerem)	Have history of kidney or respiratory problems, sleep apnea, or depression.	May interact with alcohol. High-fat meals may slow absorption of the drug. Not likely to be habit-forming.
Triazolam — a benzodiazepine derivative (Halcion)	Have a history of drug abuse, depression or respiratory conditions.	May interact with grapefruit juice, alcohol and many other medications. Can be habit-forming. Drug must be stopped gradually.
Zaleplon (Sonata)	Have severe liver impairment. Have a history of depression, liver or kidney disease, or respiratory conditions.	Can be habit-forming.
Zolpidem (Ambien)	Have a history of depression, liver or kidney disease, or respiratory conditions.	May lose effectiveness if taken for longer than two weeks.

Figure 32: Drugs That Help You Fall Asleep[54]

---

[54] Source: Micromedex.

Stage 5: Moderately Severe Cognitive Decline/Early-Stage Alzheimer's

MedicAlert + Safe Return

The Alzheimer's Association and the MedicAlert Foundation support a program called Safe Return that provides assistance to help locate a person who is lost and provides access to vital medical information in the time of need. For $49.95, with a $25 annual renewal fee, you receive an enrollment kit that includes:

- MedicAlert Identification bracelet or pendant
- Wallet card
- "6 Steps to a Safe Return" magnet
- Personal Health Record Summary
- Alzheimer's Association brochure

During stage five of Olive's care, the service was used twice and I was able to locate mother who became disoriented and lost. I would recommend the program to anyone without hesitation. Enrollment may be accomplished by phone, mail, fax or online enrolment (coming soon).

Four Easy Ways to Enroll in Safe Return

- Phone: Enroll by phone using a credit card. Call 1.888.572.8566 between 6:00 a.m. and 7:00 p.m., Monday through Friday, and 8:00 a.m. to 5:00 p.m. on Saturdays (PST). When enrolling by phone, you will be asked to provide the following information:

  Member's name and contact information

  Medical conditions

  Allergies

  Medications (including dosages)

  Member's exact wrist measurement in inches (required when ordering a bracelet)

  At least two contact names, addresses and phone numbers (more can be added if needed)

  Credit card number and expiration date

- Mail: To enroll by mail, simply print and complete the enrollment form and send with payment and the member's photo to:
  MedicAlert + Safe Return

  2323 Colorado Avenue

  Turlock, CA 95382

  You may also phone 1.888.572.8566 to have an enrollment form mailed:

  Enrollment form in English

  Enrollment form in Spanish
- Fax: Print the form, complete and fax to 1.800.863.3429.
- Online enrollment is coming soon!

Communication

Two-way verbal communication may become very strained during this stage. On occasions, you may be fortunate to have a normal conversation. Cherish these occasion for they will not last through stages six and seven. Beyond this point, it is likely the AD Loved One will not be capable of holding a thought long enough to verbalize it, especially in stage seven. Often they will eventually stop speaking.

Alzheimer's Disease Centers (ADC)

Appendix D: Alzheimer Disease Research Centers, on page 259, lists approximately thirty federally funded Alzheimer's Disease Centers (ADCs). These centers were enacted by an Act of Congress (Public Health Service Act, section 445) in 1984. The National Institute on Aging funds Alzheimer's Disease Centers (ADCs) at major medical institutions across the U.S.[55]

Researchers at these Centers are working to translate research advances

---

[55] Alzheimer's Disease Centers (ADCs) are organized under the Alzheimer's Disease Education and Referral (ADEAR) of the National, Institute of Aging, U.S. National Institutes of Health (NIH),
http://www.nia.nih.gov/Alzheimers/ResearchInformation/ResearchCenters/

Stage 5: Moderately Severe Cognitive Decline/Early-Stage Alzheimer's

into improved diagnosis and care for Alzheimer's Disease (AD) patients while, at the same time, focusing on the program's long-term goal—finding a way to cure and possibly prevent AD.

Areas of investigation range from the basic mechanisms of AD to managing the symptoms and helping families cope with the effects of the disease. Center staff conducts basic, clinical, and behavioral research and train scientists and health care providers who are new to AD research.

Although each center has its own unique area of emphasis, a common goal of the ADCs is to enhance research on AD by providing a network for sharing new ideas as well as research results. Collaborative studies draw upon the expertise of scientists from many different disciplines.

For patients and families affected by AD, the ADCs offer:

- Diagnosis and medical management (costs may vary—centers may accept Medicare, Medicaid, and private insurance).
- Information about the disease, services, and resources.
- Opportunities for volunteers to participate in drug trials, support groups, clinical research projects, and other special programs for volunteers and their families.

Some ADCs have satellite facilities which offer diagnostic and treatment services as well as research opportunities in underserved, rural, and minority communities.

My recommendation is to enter the loved one into a study group at the closest center for monitoring the progress of the disease. This can be helpful to family members and caregivers. Participation in a study group usually requires making a commitment for an autopsy upon death. The autopsy will not interfere with funeral plans. Data from the autopsy will be available to immediate family members for them to understand the cause of death and will become part of a national database at the National Alzheimer's Coordinating Center in Seattle, Washington. The Center coordinates data collection and fosters collaborative research among ADCs for seeking a treatment for the disease.

Attending Doctor

At this point, it may be necessary to change the attending doctor if they do not conduct house calls. It may not be critical at this point but it will as the disease progresses and it becomes more difficult to take the Loved One to a doctor's office for an examination. In addition, this doctor will most likely sign the death certificate. You will want to discuss the signing of the Certificate of Death with the doctor and ask him for his history signing certificates. This is an important issue since most attending doctors will list the cause of death as heart failure or pneumonia instead of Alzheimer disease. It is important that the certificate accurately indicates the cause of death as Alzheimer disease since this determines the level of research funding for the disease to seek treatment and potential cures. Additionally, the certificate of death becomes a valuable record for living decedents and for family genealogy research.

Handling Confrontations

Avoid all potential conflict from this point forward. Whatever you are feeling, anger will only complicate the care and cause you to lose valuable energy. Whatever the concern of the Loved-One, listen respectfully and go along with their wishes because in twenty minutes they will not remember the issue. If a conversation becomes confrontational, listen for the essence of the concern. Once it becomes repetitive, repeat it and then take a big deep breath. Then tell the loved one that you understand their concern and follow up with a comment like: "Let's take a walk." "Let's enjoy a glass of water." "Let's have some ice cream." This will typically diffuse the confrontation and ten minutes later the person with Alzheimer will forget the issue. This is referred as the use of a "terminal logical exactitude."[56]

---

[56] Sy Moed, who cared for his mother and sister with Alzheimer's disease and active member of Thousand Oaks Alzheimer Support Group coined this phrase., "terminal logical exactitude." An example is "Let's go have some ice cream," end of conversation.

Stage 5: Moderately Severe Cognitive Decline/Early-Stage Alzheimer's

Dementia Day Care

It is important that you are not tired from caregiving 24-hours a day, 7-days a week. You must have time for you own personal and family matters. Enrolling the loved one in a Day Care Facility for Dementia clients is an essential decision. Initially, there is usually some resistance. However, in the end it works best for the loved one and caregivers.

Join a Local Support Group

The Alzheimer Association organizes groups across the county. A local group should be located close to your home. Joining a local support group is an important aspect in the caregiving process. It is an opportunity to meet other people in similar situations, share ideas and help resolve problems. You can find a local group either through your local telephone directory, county social services organization or the internet. In addition, each district develops a local resource guide that is important to purchase, read and use as a reference.

Be aware that the Alzheimer's Support Group can provide you with a lot of benefits. However, the support groups are not a substitute for an early diagnosis. As soon as symptoms develop, review and update all legal and financial documents and develop a Caregiving Plan to withstand the tremendous stress of this disease on caregivers. The only person that is going to successfully make it through this journey alive based on your efforts is you.

Focus on You Own Health

Due to the stress of caring for a Loved One with Alzheimer's, statistically, half the caregivers either develop a significant health condition or die before the loved one. It is important to monitor your weight to insure you are near the target level for your height and age. Significant weight gains may result from the stress of the caregiving. If significant weight gain results, consider joining a group such as Weight Watchers. Also, eat nutritious food, exercise, insure your body receives adequate rest and check your vital signs regularly.

Alternative Care Options for Stages Six & Seven

Navigating through the various Federal and State entitlements for people afflicted with Alzheimer's disease is another one of the challenging and time consuming tasks. As another caregiver said, "It's a lot like playing hide-and-seek with the disadvantage of having to care for an Alzheimer patient, while at the same time you need an attorney to help you navigate and complete the application forms. It's almost like a dirty little secret the government doesn't want anyone to know about." It is difficult because the information on these programs is not easily accessible, especially over the internet. The process is time consuming to get a loved one qualified. Once qualified, Medicaid will pay for In-Home Care, or a Skilled Nursing Facility but not a Board and Care. The Board and Care facilities, for most Alzheimer patients, has superior care. Tracking billing and claims is nearly a full time activity.

Similarly, as reported January 3, 2010 by Byron Pitts on the NBC Network's, 60-Minutes, "Many veterans believe the Department of Veteran's Affairs operates under the motto of, "deny, delay, hope that you die."

Social Security Benefits

Social Security has a disability program that may be available for people with low incomes and Alzheimer's disease. However, in mother's case, even though her income from Social Security was under $900 a month, it was twelve dollars over the limit so she did not qualify for the disability program. In our case if I would have known what the criteria was for this qualification, I could have saved myself the time and effort of completing the qualification form and meeting with Social Security Personnel.

Veterans' Administration Benefits

Available to wives of deceased veterans is a little known program called, Deceased Widows Aid and Attendance Benefits from A World War II Veteran. Currently, theses benefits amount to approximately eight hundred dollars a month. Once again, you will have to meet with a Veterans Affairs (VA) Representative, complete an application and then wait for a long review to see if you are approved. Apply early and expect to be toyed with until you receive the benefits. It seems as though the VA throws up roadblocks in hopes that you will go away. If you are not satisfied with the response from the VA, SS or Medicaid, do not hesitate to contact your congressional representative. In mother's case, she died before we received any benefits.

SSDI & VA Disability Benefits-Expect an Appeal Process[57]

People applying for Social Security Disability Insurance (SSDI) benefits or Veterans Administration Disability Compensation (VADC) benefits initially expect the process to be one of meeting with representatives, completing the appropriate forms, submitting medical documentation, a scrutiny of the submitted forms, perhaps a physical examination to confirm the disability and then a fair determination by Social Security or the Veterans Administration with benefits to follow. Instead, they find that the disability process is one of rejection and a long appeal process for which they lack the expertise and especially the energy to pursue, causing a delay in the receipt of the benefits of which they are often entitled and so desperately need. Often legal assistance is required and since many disabled people are on a limited budget, hiring an attorney severely cuts into the limited income they do have. National figures show that approximately seventy percent of all initial Social Security and Veterans Administration disability claims are denied. Essential to succeeding with a social security or a veterans disability claim is retaining a law firm and an attorney specializing in VA or SS

---

[57] The author recommends reading the following books before filing SSDI or VA Disability Claims:
Nolo's Guide to Social Security Disability, 4th Edition by David A. Morton III, Published by NOLO, May 2008, 492page paperback, ISBN-13: 9781413307641 and ISBN: 1413307647.
The The Veteran's Survival Guide: How to File and Collect on VA Claims, Second Edition by John D. Roche, Potomac Books, Inc., November 2006, 304 page paperback, ISBN-13: 9781597970518 and ISBN: 1597970514, and
Claim Denied!: How to Appeal a VA Denial of Benefits by John D. Roche, Potomac Books Inc., December 31, 2008, 210 page paperback ISBN-10: 1597971162 and ISBN-13: 978-1597971164.

disabilities benefits to assist with the claim.

The following is a suggested process which may improve the acceptance of your initial claim or help an appeal be successful so you may begin receiving disability benefits:

- Fully document and describe your condition and symptoms to your doctor(s).

- Do not apply for benefits until you have all the current medical documents available to support your claim from private doctor(s) and laboratories. This recommendation is made since once you file the claim it will establish time limits for completion.

- Submit all forms with cover letter outlining the documents included in the mailing. At the top of each page list your name, page # of total pages, subject, claim number, file number (which is usually your social security number), date mailed, and certified mail receipt number. Mail the document via U.S. Postal Service certified mail with return receipt requested. Follow-up 10-days later by going to the U.S. Postal Service internet site or post office and obtain the U.S. Postal Delivery Tracking & Confirmation Report and file the document in your three ring binder.

- When there is a meeting or phone call, afterward summarize the conversation in a letter and mail the document certified mail with a return receipt requested.

- Keep all the documents regarding the disability in a 3-ring binder. At the very front of the binder, keep a log of all contacts. The log should be organized in reverse chronological order with the last activity listed first. The log should be organized with the following column headings: date, day and approximate time; investigation/action item; initiated by & person responsible for action item; person contact & position; results, comments or additional information; and follow-up date. If the person is not willing to provide you their last name, ask for their organization employee number.

Stage 5: Moderately Severe Cognitive Decline/Early-Stage Alzheimer's

- Obtain copies of lab test results and documentation from your doctor describing the disorder or impairment. If you have trouble obtaining this information, cite the "Freedom of Information Act" and threaten legal action if the documents are not released to you in a timely and complete manner.
- If your initial application is denied, appeal within 30 days.
- Understand that most initial applications are denied and don't let this negatively interfere with your positive attitude or emotions.
- Do not give up. The SSA and VA deny initial claims because theoretically it saves the organizations money and makes the organizations look good financially and well managed. In reality it ends up costing the government and taxpayers more money in the long run as the untreated condition deteriorates because of the person's lack of financial resources. In the end the situation results in increased Medicare and Medicaid expenses because of the neglected health problem.
- Keep appealing in a timely and succinct fashion when denied and be positive.
- Follow doctor's orders. Take necessary medical prescriptions, rehabilitation, etc.
- Make thorough notes and keep an organized file of all records.
- Know the facts of your case and handling of similar claims.
- Be prepared to discuss your case at any time.
- Be patient with the process, even with an attorney the process takes time, maybe as much as three years.

In the case of VA disabilities you may be assisted in filing a claim by a service organization such as the Disabled American Veterans, American Legion or Veterans of Foreign Wars. The process for filing a claim is as follows:

- File an initial application with your regional VA office. You will then get what is called a Ratings Decision.

- If you are not satisfied with the outcome, then file a notice of disagreement to your regional office within one year. You will then get a Statement of the Case (SOC).
- At this point you may submit additional evidence. Then you will get a Supplemental Statement of the Case (SSOC).
- If you are still not satisfied with the decision, you can appeal to the Board of Veterans Appeals (BVA). You do this at your regional office. You have 60 days from your SOC or one year from the Rating Decision. You have an opportunity for a hearing before the BVA at this stage. You will then receive your decision from the BVA. This can take a very long time. The BVA can do a few things. They may send it back on remand to the RO for a new decision. They can also grant benefits. Remand (court procedure) is an action by an appellate court in which it remands, sends back, a case to the trial court or lower appellate court for action.
- Lastly, the RO can issue the final denial of the BVA. If you are still unhappy with the decision, you can file suit at the United States Court of Appeals for Veterans Claims or the CAVC. You have 120 days from the BVA decision to file an appeal.

Medicaid Long Term Care Benefit

Medicaid is a federal program typically administered by each state's welfare agency. It is important to deal with the long-term care division as opposed to the group that deals exclusively with low, limited income families. Eligibility and benefits vary from state to state. The program is typically administered by a state welfare agency. In each state, the program usually has a unique name. Medicaid covers all or a portion of nursing home costs. People with Alzheimer's can qualify for long-term care only if they have minimal income and cash assets.

Once again, you will have to meet with a representative, complete a qualification form and wait to see if your loved one qualifies for Medicaid Long Term Care. In-home care and skilled nursing facilities are covered under Medicaid. The following is the typical criteria for qualification in

Stage 5: Moderately Severe Cognitive Decline/Early-Stage Alzheimer's

2008:

Financial Qualification Criteria (Partial List)
- Monthly Income less than $1911
- Resources amounting to less than $2000 (couples $3000)

Exempt Resources:
- Home in which applicant, spouse or dependent child resides; or to which applicant intends to return with an equity value of less than $500,000.
- One car
- Personal (clothing and furniture) belongings
- Term life insurance
- Irrevocable burial policy

Resources That Count:
- Checking and savings accounts
- Stocks, bonds, investments, annuities
- Rental property/land, vacation homes
- Recreational vehicles
- Whole life insurance and revocable burial policies

If a married applicant has more than $2,000 in resources, the spouse may be eligible for spousal protection, but may need to spend down resources. An applicant with more than $1,911 in monthly income may need a Medicaid Qualifying Trust.

An Income or Medicaid Qualifying Trust provides a means for individuals with a monthly income greater than $1911 in 2008 to receive Medicaid assistance with the cost of nursing home care or home care. To qualify, the individual must have resources of less than $2000 (couples $3000) and income less than $5,546 per month.

Recovery
The Medicaid Estate Recovery Act is a federally mandated program designed to help recover all Medicaid costs from the estates of individuals who own property and who receive Medicaid. All payments made by

Medicaid including: provider reimbursement and cost sharing for Medicare and private insurance coverage (Part B Medicare premiums, co-insurance or co-payments for Medicare services, and deductibles for Medicare Part A and B) may be recovered.

The following estates (homes or other real property) are exempt:
- If the individual is survived by the spouse, a child under 21, or a blind or disabled dependent;
- If there is a brother or sister who lived in the home for at least a year before the individual went to a nursing home and has lived there continuously or
- If a son or daughter lived in the house for at least two years before the deceased entered a nursing home, thus allowing the parent to delay entry into a nursing home, and if the son or daughter has continued to live in the home since the parent entered a nursing home.

This program has a three-year look-back at asset ownership for qualification. Mother qualified for this program. However, I could not find immediate availability among the twenty nursing homes I evaluated. None compared to the quality of care mother was receiving at a Board & Care, which is not covered by this benefit but should be. Most of the time a Board &Care Facility or Assisted Living Facility is less expensive than a nursing home.

Applying for Medicaid
In California the program is called Medi-Cal and there currently is a single form, MC 210 10/07 APPLICATION which you may complete online or download and mail-in.[58]

---

[58] This form may be found on the internet at: http://www.dhcs.ca.gov/services/medi-cal/Documents/PDF_Medi-Cal%20Applications/English/English%20Application.pdf. See also, http://www.dhcs.ca.gov/services/medi-cal/Pages/MediCalApplications.aspx.

Stage 5: Moderately Severe Cognitive Decline/Early-Stage Alzheimer's

Care Alternatives

The following is an important consideration in the alternative you choose. "More than one of every two (55 percent) Alzheimer's disease patients residing in the community in northern California had severe cognitive impairments, compared with more than nine of every ten institutionalized patients (94 percent). One of five community-resident patients needed assistance with inside mobility (25%), compared with seven of ten institutionalized patients (70%), and almost all institutionalized patients required assistance with dressing, grooming, bathing, and using the toilet. These findings indicate that the nursing home is the caregiver of last resort for persons with Alzheimer's disease, because very few patients were institutionalized unless they had significant cognitive and functional impairments."[59]

In-Home Care

Assuming the afflicted is qualified, Medicaid will cover the cost of in-home care including a live-in caregiver. The disadvantage is the paperwork that needs to be maintained by the primary caregiver. Personally, I feel this should be the preferred option for a person afflicted with Alzheimer as long as the primary caregiver is in good health and can handle the management of the situation. Not everyone can handle the stress that this kind of a situation can place on the individual.

Board & Care Homes

Other than their own home, Board & Care Facilities are the best place for an Alzheimer patient because they are small facilities resembling a home with a maximum of seven clients at each location. My opinion is the care is

---

[59] Dorothy Rice, Patrick Fox, Wendy Max, and Pamela Webber are affiliated with the Institute for Health and Aging, University of California, San Francisco (UCSF), School of Nursing. David Lindeman and Ernestine Segura are affiliated with the Alzheimer's Disease Center at the University of California, Davis. Walter Hauck is on the faculty of the Department of Epidemiology and Biostatistics at the UCSF School of Medicine. The study titled "Economic Burden of Alzheimer's Disease Care," is published in Health Affairs, Volume 12, Issue 2, 164-176.

superior to a skill nursing facility. However, because of lobbying efforts of Skilled Nursing Facility Corporations who own most large facilities, Medicaid currently will only pay for skilled nursing facilities.

Skilled Nursing

The first problem with a skilled nursing facility is usually availability. This is the case since only a limited number of beds are reserved for Medicaid Pay clients. The second issue is the quality of the care, which is usually substantially lower than a Board & Care. It is surprising to me that the government does not realize the value of board and care and include them in reimbursement. Instead, the government pays a higher cost at skilled nursing facilities and the quality of the care is often marginal. The quality of care is usually lower because of high turnover due to low wages, understaffing and the use of old poorly maintained facilities.

Board & Care vs Skilled Nursing Facility[60]

Many nursing homes are aging and the industry has suffered through so many scandals involving patient care, that many elderly shun the thought of entering such institutions. A 2003 survey by the AARP, an advocacy group for older Americans, found that just 1% of Americans over fifty with a disability wanted to move to a nursing home. Most people at age eighty-five do not want to spend their final days sitting in the hallway of an Alzheimer's Wing of a traditional nursing home while patients yell at each other or are drugged into a stupor with anti-psychotic drugs so they maybe efficiently managed. Figure 33 on page 126 is an analysis of a Skilled Nursing Facility and Board & Care Home Comparison.

Selecting Care Facility

The key to find an appropriate care facility is:

---

[60] See Wall Street Journal Artitle titled, "Rising Challenger Takes on Elder-Care System," front page, A1, June 24, 2008 and Robet Wood Johnson Foundation internet site regarding their investment in "Green Houses."

Stage 5: Moderately Severe Cognitive Decline/Early-Stage Alzheimer's

- Should be close to the primary caregiver's home to make frequent visits convenient.
- Loved one is kept safe, clean and provided adequate nutrition, exercise and rest.

	SKILLED NURSING FACILITY	BOARD & CARE HOME
General Ambience	Institution	Homelike Feel
Typical Number of Clients	Usually 100 or 200	ten or less
Caregiver to Patient Ratio	1:20	1 or 2:7 during daytime, 1:7 at night
Patient Care/Lifestyle	Often rigid, impersonal and at times degrading life	"Patient-centered" Flexible, personal and more humane care.
Provide Skilled Nursing	Yes, One or two RNs on duty 24-Hours/Day	No, unless on Hospice. Maybe contracted with Separate external service.
Care for Patient with Stage 3 or 4 Bed Sores or On an IV or Breathing Tube	Yes	No

Figure 33: Board & Care vs Skilled Nursing Facility

Figure 33 above Compares Skilled Nursing Facilities to Board & Care Homes (B&C). Most caregivers prefer to place their loved one in Board & Care Facilities because of the quality, personalized care and homelike ambience. If funds are limited, a skilled nursing facility is usually the only viable choice. A form is on page 196 to help you choose between available alternatives.

Hospice Care

Hospice care is intended palliative care during the last six month of life. It is covered by Medicare. At six month intervals the person will need to be requalified for Hospice care. Requalification criteria vary by state but often must include the following for dementia due to Alzheimer's disease and related disorders:

Stage 5: Moderately Severe Cognitive Decline/Early-Stage Alzheimer's

- Stage seven or beyond according to the Functional Assessment Staging Test (FAST) scale
- Unable to ambulate without assistance
- Unable to dress without assistance
- Unable to bathe without assistance
- Urinary and fecal incontinence (intermittent or constant)
- No consistent meaningful verbal communication: stereotypical phrases only or the ability to speak is limited to six or fewer intelligent words.

For a look at the forms often used in the evaluation, see Appendix G: Extended Hospice Patient Re-qualification, on page 284.

Placement in Independent Care

We discussed placement in independent care earlier in the chapter. You may want to go back and review the information presented in this section on Placement, on page 101 of this book. The decision to place a Loved-One in an independent care facility will be one of the most challenging decisions you will make in your life. For each person the timing will be different. It is ultimately dependant on your own health, tolerance level and other individual criteria. The Board & Care/Nursing Home Evaluation on page 196 is included to facilitate this decision.

Stage 6

Stage 6: Severe Cognitive & Functional Decline/Moderately Severe or Mid-Stage Alzheimer's

Typical at Stage 6: [61] Memory difficulties continue to worsen, significant personality changes may emerge and affected individuals need extensive help with customary daily activities. At this stage individuals may:

- Lose most awareness of recent experiences and events as well as awareness of their surroundings
- Recollect their personal history imperfectly, although they generally recall their own name
- Occasionally forget the name of their spouse or primary caregiver but generally can distinguish familiar from unfamiliar faces
- Need help getting dressed properly without supervision, may make such errors as putting pajamas over daytime clothes or shoes on wrong feet
- Experience disruption of their normal sleep/waking cycle

---

[61] The Alzheimer Association Internet Site, September 2007, Alzheimer's Association National Office 225 N. Michigan Ave., Fl. 17, Chicago, IL 60601 or http://www.alz.org.

Stage 6: Severe Cognitive & Functional Decline/Moderately Severe or Mid-Stage Alzheimer's

- **Need help with handling details of toileting (flushing toilet, wiping and disposing of tissue properly)**
- **Have increasing episodes of urinary or fecal incontinence**
- **Experience significant personality changes and behavioral symptoms, including suspiciousness and delusions (for example, believing that their caregiver is an impostor); hallucinations (seeing or hearing things that are not really there); or compulsive, repetitive behaviors such as hand-wringing or tissue shredding**
- **Tend to wander and become lost**

Stage 6: Caregiving - Less Physically Demanding More Emotionally Stressful

Figure 34 on page 130 is a picture of mother one month before admission to Leisure Living Board and Care (LLB&C) in Agoura Hills, California. Wednesday, November 10, 2004, I drove mother five miles and admitted her to Leisure Living Board and Care (LLB&C). Mother was still able to walk on her own at this point, had a good appetite and could carry on limited conversation. Mother continued to be positive about living as she had been her entire life.

The staff asked me to initially stay away if I could for three weeks to give mother time to acclimate to her new surroundings. Three weeks later on a Friday night, I visited mother just after she had finished eating dinner. I walked up to mother, gave her a big hug and a kiss on the cheek. Mother immediately said, "Hello Bob, how have you been?" I said, "I am fine. How are you doing?" Mother then asked, "Bob, have we done a lot of remodeling?" I asked, "Why." Mother said, "Well, everything looks so fresh and cheery." I said, "Yes, mother things do look nice." Mother then asked the man who was preparing food to come over to the table. Mother said, "Bob, this is my new helper, he prepares really delicious meals." Mother continued to walk in the back yard, eat nutritious food and began to rest longer.

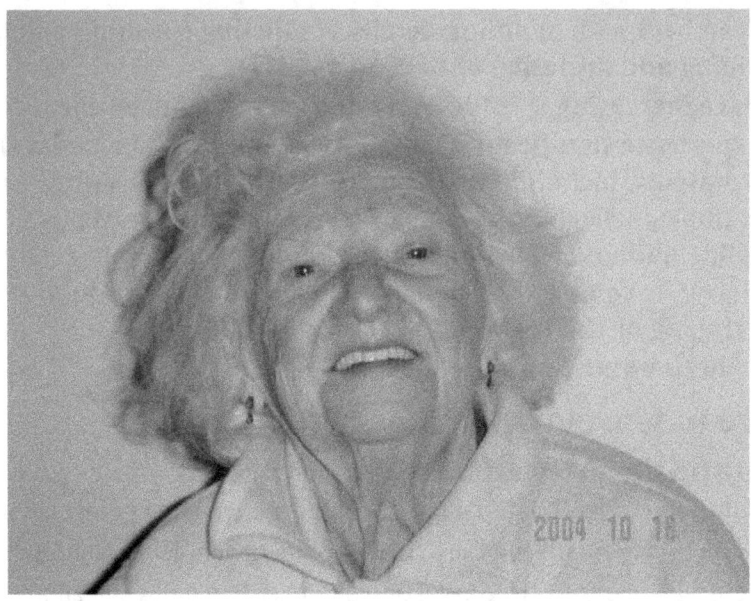

Figure 34: Olive at Bob's Home, October 16, 2004

During December 2004 I took mother, along with the aid of a caregiver from LLB&C, to Olive's doctor's office for a periodic general examination. The doctor was once a neighbor and our daughters were on the same baseball teams when they were young. It was very difficult getting mother from Leisure Living into the car and then into the doctor's office and then return to LLB&C. As soon as we arrived at the doctor's office, mother had to go to the bathroom, then again and again for the second and third time. Then after she was in the examining room, she had to go three more times. Finally, the doctor entered the room and as soon as he began to examine mother, she had to go to the bathroom again. The doctor motioned to me to come to his office where he asked, "How are you, Bob." I said, "I am fine." The doctor then proceeded to tell me, "I have been through this with both of my sets of parents. Your mother is suffering from anxiety. I will prescribe a medication for your mother's anxiety so she sleeps well at night and for her Alzheimer disease but this is a very difficult stage. Whatever I prescribe will only work for a short time if at all and then we will have to try something else. This is very difficult. I don't want you to lose confidence in me during the process." I thanked the doctor and we went back into the examining room where he completed the examination. Afterward we drove along the lake, stopped for ice cream and then returned to Leisure Living.

Later during December 2004, I also visited the same doctor and found out that the results from my PSA Test were on the high side at 6.4. Since the PSA had even been much higher, as high as fourteen, during the last four years, there seemed to be no cause for alarm.

Figure 35: Christmas Celebration, Leisure Living Board & Care (LLB&C), Agoura Hills, CA, December 16, 2004 on page 132 and Figure 36: Olive and Ken Bayus at LLB&C, December 26, 2004 on page 133 were the last enjoyable, joyous holiday occasions. Early in 2005, mother continued her decline at a more rapid pace.

In March 2005 I drove from California to Wisconsin to begin to prepare our home for sale. I grew-up in this home that my parents built with the assistance of family members. I found this to be another of many emotionally draining tasks that needed to be completed. As soon as I began the preparation, I noticed notes for me that mother had placed in a bible, in photo albums, on pictures, in her jewelry box and other places. Reading these notes was a very emotionally disturbing experience. They all started, "Bob, if something happens to me . . . ."

When I had returned to Wisconsin during late December 1997 to take Olive to The Mayo Clinic to see if she would tolerate some medication for her heart, I had filled the freezer food for her to eat. Now, in the process of preparing the house for sale, during the spring 2005, I found all the meat that I had purchased for mother in December 1997 still all in the freezer. The meat had been in there for seven years. Never in my life did I ever expect to have to sell either the lakeside cottage or the home where I was raised. For the last twenty years, I had always planned upon retirement at age sixty-six and dividing my time between Wisconsin and California.

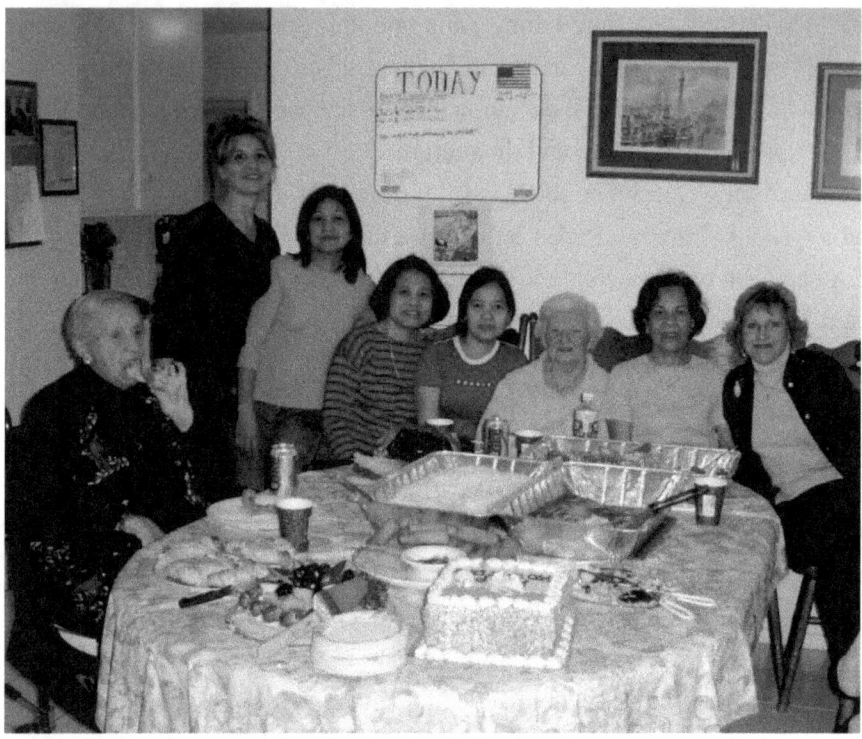

Figure 35: Christmas Celebration, Leisure Living Board & Care (LLB&C), Agoura Hills, CA, December 16, 2004

One day in April 2005 I visited mother at the LLB&C. There were more than the usual number of people at the facility that day. Mother said, "I'm scared." I asked her, "What scares you mother?" Mother repeated, "I think they are going to move me to a nursing home." I asked mother, "What makes you think that?" Mother replied, "Because of all the people that are in the house." I responded to mother, "They are not moving you anywhere. Mother, you are going to continue to live right here in this house." Mother said, "O! Good, Bob" and sighed with relief.

Stage 6: Severe Cognitive & Functional Decline/Moderately Severe or Mid-Stage Alzheimer's

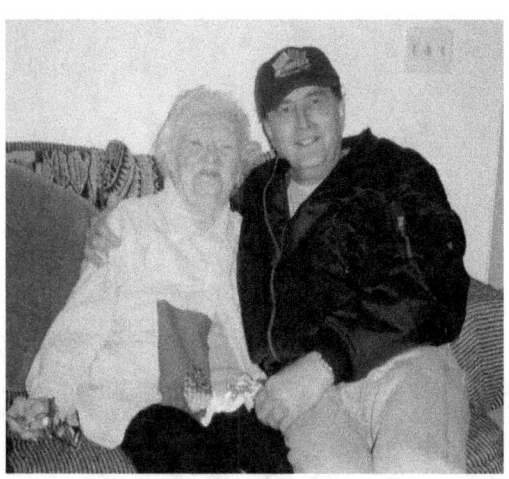

Figure 36: Olive and Ken Bayus at LLB&C, December 26, 2004

May 2005, I returned to California from Wisconsin to check on mother and attend my daughter Shelby's college graduation in June. Mother's mental condition had continued to deteriorate and she was beginning to experience walking problems when she was on her own without her cane. Figure 37: Olive and son, Bob at LLB&C, May 19, 2005 on page 134 was a photo taken on one of the many visits during this time. You can see in the picture how frail mother had become and needed to lean against me for balance. In May 2005, I changed local doctors to one who did house calls. The new doctor examined mother at Leisure Living. The examination went smoothly and except for her Alzheimer's, Olive's vital signs were normal.

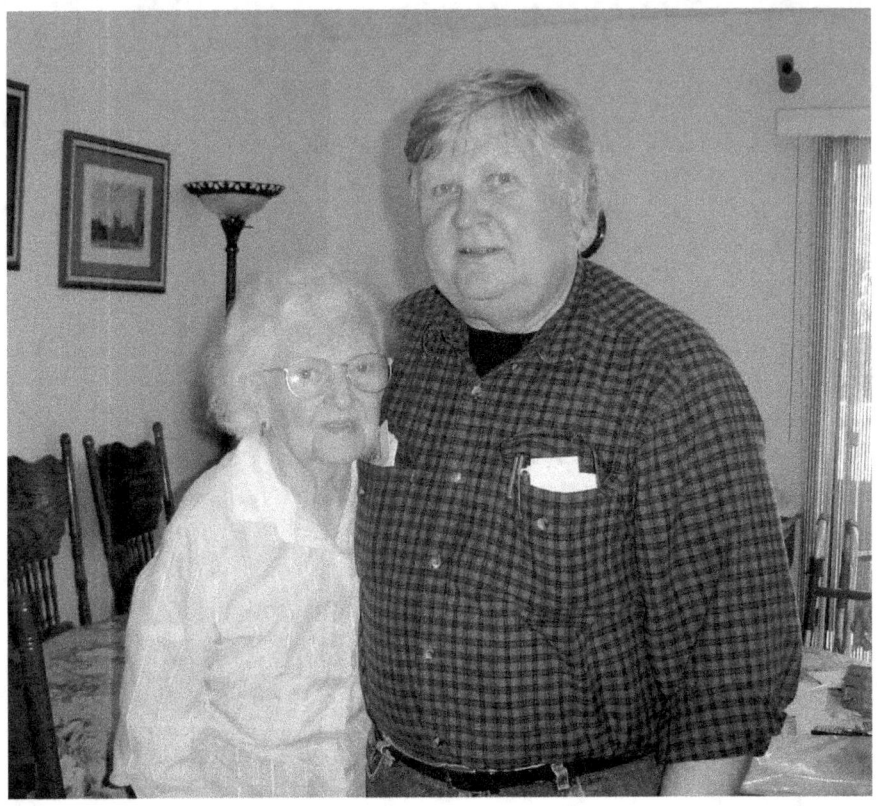

Figure 37: Olive and son, Bob at LLB&C, May 19, 2005

Mother's health continued to decline significantly during the spring and summer of 2005. While I was preparing our home for sale in Wisconsin, friends Roger and Alice visited mother weekly. During this time, they were concerned that mother would not survive until I returned. During October/November 2005 there was a rapid decline in mother's health. During this time, she stopped walking and her speech became limited to three or four words. This occurred because Olive could not hold a thought long enough for her to verbalize it. I personally found this very stressful in attempting to communicate with mother. I felt so helpless on these visits to see her suffer.

When I was in Wisconsin in July 2005, I suffered a heat stroke on Friday,

Stage 6: Severe Cognitive & Functional Decline/Moderately Severe or Mid-Stage Alzheimer's

July 1st, spent four hours at the hospital and then rested at home for the long Fourth of July weekend. Also, during this month I noticed that my own energy had declined significantly since the beginning of the year.

During October/November 2005 mother entered the final stage seven of the disease. This is the stage when individuals lose their functional ability to respond to their environment, the ability to walk, to speak and the ability to control movement.

During October/November 2005, Olive stopped walking and by December was confined to a wheel chair. At the same time mother would get a thought in her mind and could only verbalize three to five words before losing her train of thought. By late 2006 Olive would get a thought and just make garbled sounds. The frustration mother was experiencing at this time was very difficult to witness. Starting during this period she spent her day sitting in a recliner between the kitchen and dining area. From this position mother could watch the staff prepare food in the kitchen and enjoy the aroma of the food cooking. Additionally, Olive could look into the mirrored refrigerator door and view the beautiful backyard with flowers, trees with bird feeders hanging from the branches and mountains in the distance. Once, a roadrunner even strutted across the back yard. It is the only time we noticed a roadrunner in California.

During November 2005, her house was sold. Late November 2005, I moved some of the contents from Wisconsin to California and placed them in storage for Olive's granddaughters and my own home. Selling the house and distributing the contents was a sad ending to another chapter of my life. Having lived through the Great Depression mother and dad were very frugal, saving a lot of unnecessary things (screws, nails, canning jars, old televisions, Christmas decorations, chairs, etc.) for rainy days which never came and needed to be discarded. I took a lot of these items to the nearby Goodwill Store. Additionally, I filled a forty foot disposal container to the top. A visit with mother upon my return from Wisconsin is shown in Figure 38: Olive and son, Bob, Leisure Living, November 19, 2005 on page 136.

Upon returning from Wisconsin, I visited mother at Leisure Living and could see the drastic change in her appearance. A comparison of the picture taken in May 2005 with the picture from November of the same year shows the significant changes that she was experiencing. She is much more frail and the expression on her face is one of emptiness.

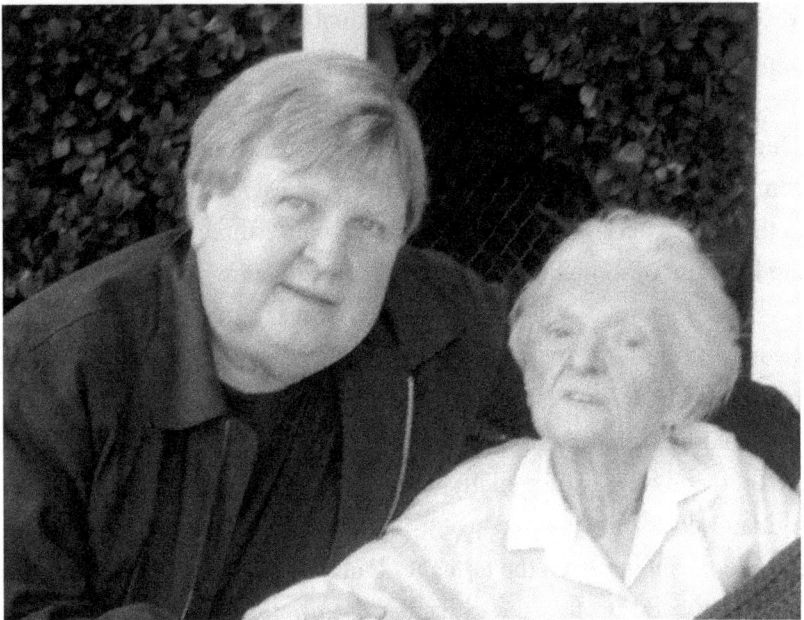

Figure 38: Olive and son, Bob, Leisure Living, November 19, 2005

December 2005, I flew back to Wisconsin to pick-up Olive's Buick that was in the garage for repairs and then drove on to The Mayo Clinic. At The Mayo Clinic, I checked in to find out why my energy had declined so significantly along with a host of other health concerns. The day before Christmas Eve 2005, The Mayo Clinic called at eight o'clock in the evening and said, "The biopsy results are back from the lab and your tests results are positive for cancer. Make arrangements to return to The Mayo Clinic as early as you can in 2006 for treatment, have a Merry Christmas."

Before the LLB&C Christmas Party 2005, I invited Sue Lindeman, Facilitator for the local Alzheimer Support, and Roger and Alice Eisele to come to my home and help educate my daughters, Aubrey and Shelby, about

Stage 6: Severe Cognitive & Functional Decline/Moderately Severe or Mid-Stage Alzheimer's

their grandmother's Alzheimer's disease. My ex-wife Nina and friend Ken Bayus joined us. I felt my daughters needed to have this discussion to prepare them for the changes they were going to experience with their grandmother at Christmas. Sue had lost her husband to the disease and Alice Eisele had lost her first husband to the disease when he was only fifty-seven. Roger Eisele lost his father to the disease and was currently caring for his mother, Grace, who had also been diagnosed with Alzheimer's. Sue, Alice and Roger had a nice informative conversation with Aubrey and Shelby describing the disease to them and answering their questions. Afterwards we all went to the LLB&C Christmas festivities. Alice who had worked at Senior Concerns even got Olive to dance briefly.

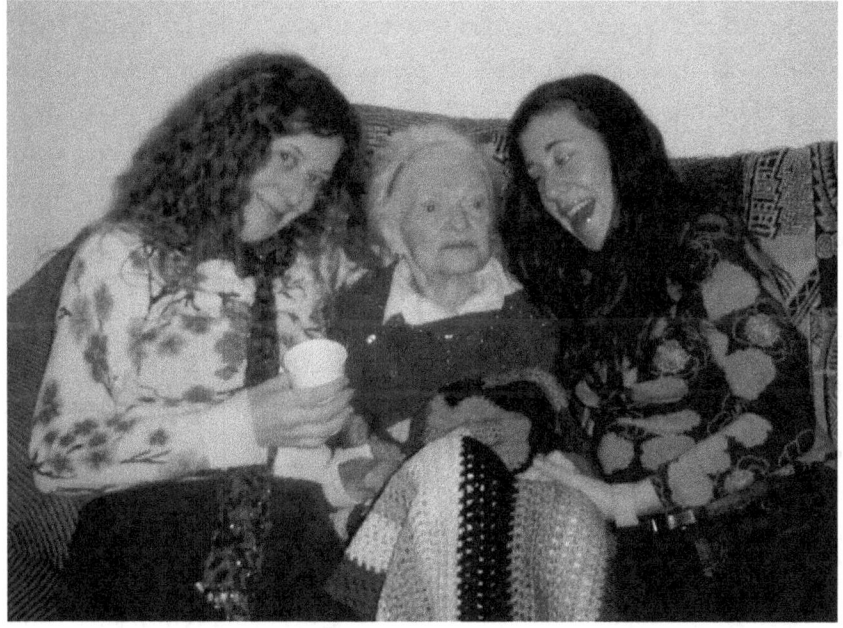

Figure 39: Granddaughters Shelby & Aubrey & Olive, LLB&C, December 16, 2005

Alzheimer's--What My Mother's Caregiving Taught Me

Early 2006 I returned to The Mayo Clinic for additional testing and subsequent cancer surgery.

The Friday before the surgery Shelby and I drove from The Mayo Clinic in Rochester, MN to Lauderdale Lakes and walked out on the frozen Middle Lake. Shelby turned to me and said dad, "I don't understand why you had to sell grandma's house. Why this place is absolutely gorgeous. That is, unless you had to!" By this time Alzheimer's used up every single asset that my parents worked for so diligently their entire lives. It was now gone. All that remains are the memories.

On Tuesday, February 14, 2006 as I was in the surgical suite about to be anesthetized for the surgery, LLB&C called and said, "Your mother has been rushed to the hospital because of pneumonia. We know you are about to undergo cancer surgery and a "Do Not Resuscitate Order" is in place (see Do Not Resuscitate Orders (DNRO), on page 235). We just want to double check with you and see what kind of life support you want Olive to receive." I indicated, "Have the doctors do what is necessary to keep her alive until I return to California." The cancer surgery was long and I lost a lot of blood during the operation. Fifteen days later I received the news that "minimal cancer cells were detected in follow-up testing." At least there was some good news to lessen my anxiety.

I returned to California in mid March exhausted. My friend Ken was waiting to drive me home from the airport. After a week of rest, I began visiting mother regularly once again. Ken drove a hundred thirty miles nearly every weekend to help me out and visit mother. Ken and my neighbor John were very important resources in my recovery from the cancer surgery and in maintaining my spirits.

During June 2006, I returned to The Mayo Clinic for follow-up testing. The test indicated the surgery was successful with a small number of residual cancer cells. I returned to California fairly free of cancer cells, but with all kinds of aches and pains that made it difficult to sleep for more than an hour or two at a time, resulting in constant fatigue.

Stage 6: Recommendation for Caregivers

An Alzheimer's Patients Wish

The following poem was written by an unknown poet. You should use this poem to guide your care through stages six and seven:

Do not ask me to remember.
Don't try to make me understand.
Let me rest and know you're with me.
Kiss my cheek and hold my hand.

I am confused beyond your concept.
I am sad, sick, and lost.
All I know is that I need you
To be with me at all cost.

Do not lose your patience with me.
Do not scold or curse or cry.
I cannot help the way I am acting,
I can't be different 'though I try.

Just remember that I need you,
That the best of me is gone.
Please do not fail to stand beside me,
Love me 'til my life is done.

Figure 40: Poem, "An Alzheimer's Patients Wish"

Caregiver Health - Focus on Extreme Physical & Mental Endurance

To deal with the stress the disease causes at this stage, focus on your own nutrition, exercise and rest. You may want to take a walk in your neighborhood or read a book before you go to bed to get your mind off your care and concern for your loved one.

Time Together

Time together during this phase may become strained as cognitive decline continues and functional decline makes caregiving difficult. The Alzheimer patient's attention span may become short at the end of this phase. A thought may be difficult for them to verbalize. Touch and other nonverbal methods of communication become very important in this phase. Give the loved one a hug upon arrival and departure and hold the loved one's hand during much of the visit.

Stage 7

Stage 7: Very Severe Cognitive, Functional & Behavioral Decline/Severe Late-Stage Alzheimer's

Typical at Stage 7: [62]

- **This is the final stage of the disease when individuals lose the ability to respond to their environment, the ability to speak and, ultimately, the ability to control movement**
- **Frequently, individuals lose their capacity for recognizable speech, although words or phrases may occasionally be uttered**
- **Individuals need help with eating and toileting and there is general incontinence of urine**
- **Individuals lose the ability to walk without assistance, then the ability to sit without support, the ability to smile, and the ability to hold their head up. Reflexes become abnormal and muscles grow rigid. Swallowing is impaired**

---

[62] The Alzheimer Association Internet Site, September 2007, Alzheimer's Association National Office 225 N. Michigan Ave., Fl. 17, Chicago, IL 60601 or http://www.alz.org.

Stage 7: Caregiving - Very Draining Emotionally

During March 2006, a third doctor came to check on mother, take her blood pressure, heart rate and talk with Olive. The previous doctor had moved his practice to another city since the last examination. The third doctor introduced himself and asked, "Olive, how do you feel?" Mother responded, "Pretty good." The doctor continued, "Is anything hurting you?" Mother replied, "No." The doctor then asked mother, "Do you usually feel happy or sad?" Mother was silent for a while and clearly said, "I'm sad." The doctor then asked, "Why are you feeling sad?" Mother eyes grew large, her facial expression became sad as tears developed in the corner of her eyes and then ran down her cheeks. She took a deep breath. The doctor then said, "Ok Olive, I am going to finish examining you, is that ok." Mother nodded, ok. A few minutes later Olive said as she did frequently, "Help me." Olive began this behavior during the last year, whereby she would constantly repeat "Help me" over and over. The doctor then asked mother, "How can I help you Olive?" There was no response from Mother. This was mother's usual reply. Later the doctor indicated mother had continued to decline since the last visit but basically was ok and holding her own.

In May 2006 I asked a lifelong friend Sam, who is a pastor, to visit mother because I did not feel she would live long. Sam had a full calendar at this time and was not able to visit until late June (see photos on page 143). I asked Sam to read Olive some scriptures and offer her communion. I felt mother would enjoy both. Instead, when Sam said, "Do you remember me Olive?" Mother said, "No." Sam proceed to tell mother, "I am a Lutheran minister and came to visit you and see if you want me to read you some scriptures from the bible or give you communion." Mother's reply was, "No, I'm Methodist." Three years earlier Sam invited Olive and me to his church on Mother's Day. Before the sermon, Sam asked Olive to stand and he introduced her to the members of his church. Sam said to Olive and the entire congregation, "Olive, I want you to know, you have been a very

Stage 7: Very Severe Cognitive, Functional & Behavioral Decline/Severe Late-Stage Alzheimer's

important person in my life, especially while I was growing up in grade school and high school, as well as now, as an adult, parent and a pastor." Sam then based his sermon on some thoughtful observations he made of Olive's life as he was growing up including some humorous incidents. Afterwards we went to Sam's home where Sam's wife Ellen had prepared a delicious lunch. Sam made this one of the best Mother's Days in Olive's life.

Christmas 2006 was a sad time. Mother's condition had declined severely. I thought this would be Olive's last Christmas. At this point Olive could no longer walk or talk and required assistance in all her daily activities. The atmosphere at LLB&C was festive with holiday decorations everywhere but I don't think my mother was even aware that it was the Christmas season. Between Christmas and New Years, a professional singer gave a concert singing traditional Christmas songs. Off and on mother would yell out. I gently asked mother to please be quiet but she continued her outbursts. Finally, my oldest daughter Aubrey, who is a kindergarten teacher, and I switched seats. Aubrey, in her caring manner was able to quiet mother's emotions. During the performance, I think mother was having a problem dealing with all the stimulation of the lights, sound and people.

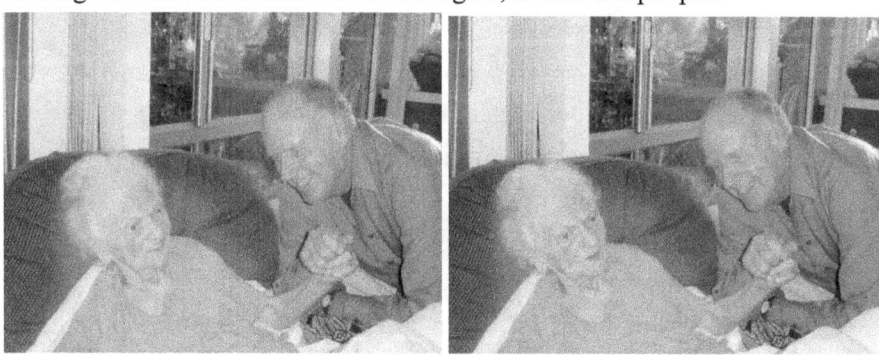

Figure 41: Olive & Lifelong Friend & Pastor, Sam Platts at LLB&C, June 27, 2006

Alzheimer's--What My Mother's Caregiving Taught Me

In the two pictures on page 143 of Olive and Sam Platts, Olive looks confused and terrified. The pictures also show that she has lost a significant amount of weight. However, she gained the weight back during the fall of 2006 and spring of 2007. In Figure 42: Olive in Leisure Living Back Yard, June 2007 on page 145, it is apparent that Olive gained back some of the weight she lost a year earlier and looks much healthier. In early May 2007, Olive began receiving Morphine (Roxanol®) for pain and Seroquel for anxiety. At the same time she was taken off all her heart arrhythmia and anti-hypertension medication. The result of taking her off these medications caused no change in her vital signs.

During March/April 2007, the pain from my cancer surgery intensified to a peak. After I returned from the May Clinic in June 2006, musculoskeletal pain especially in my shoulders increased significantly. The pain was so severe that I could only sleep for a few hours at a time in any position and the pain would awaken me. Then I would seek another tolerable position to rest. I was tired twenty-four hours a day during this period. I was certain I was going to die so during April 2007, I began writing letters to friends and stored them on my computer in a shared public folder. I am sure the stress from dealing with my mother's declining health was contributing to the extreme pain I was experiencing.

During March 2007, I met with Hospice to have mother taken off the anti-psychotic medication, Haldol. I felt the Haldol was making mother's behavioral condition worse. The medication seemed to cause mother to yell and scream, hear noises and think that other people were bothering her. Finally, the medication was changed to Seroquel and mother's behavior improved significantly.

In April/May 2007, I met with Hospice again because mother had been on Hospice for 12-months and they were considering taking her off the service. This did not make any sense to me because mother could not walk, talk, was incontinent and needed help with all her daily needs. Finally, after spending a considerable number of days researching the topic on the internet, I found the criteria for requalification, met with Hospice and they agreed to requalify

Stage 7: Very Severe Cognitive, Functional & Behavioral Decline/Severe Late-Stage Alzheimer's

mother for another six-months. There is a list of the criteria in Appendix G: Extended Hospice Patient Re-qualification, beginning on page 284.

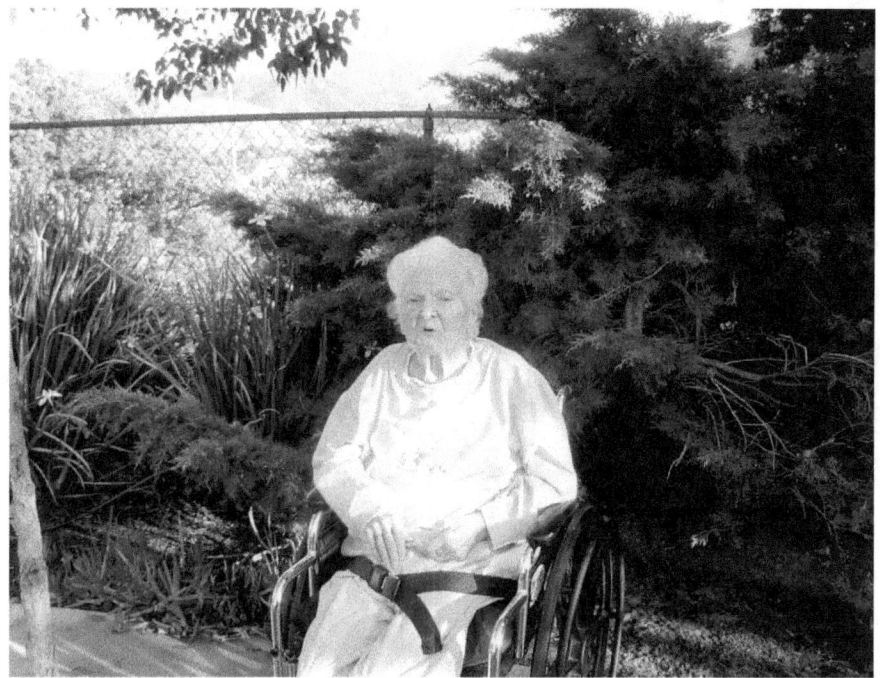

Figure 42: Olive in Leisure Living Back Yard, June 2007

During a visit in June 2007, I sat down with mother, comforted her and then read from some notes on index cards I had previously prepared. I told her that she had been fortunate to enjoy such a good life. I had made the same comments on Mother's Day and on several other occasions during the previous six months. In detail, I read from my notes, "Mother, you have been a special person in my life and I want to thank you for everything you have done for me. You have had a full life with all your friends and relatives, everyone has appreciated the delicious meals you always prepared and the many beautiful oil paintings you completed. You have had a long, full life. Mother I love you and I want to thank you for everything you have done for me." Mother looked up at me, smiled and threw me three quick kisses. Afterwards I pushed mother around the backyard in her wheel chair. This was the last time I saw mother smile. Near her birthday on August 5th, Olive lost her ability to hold her head up. On the day of her birthday, she simply stared at the floor and would not look up, eat or say anything. Five days before mother's death she started the dying processes. At 10:45 pm on Wednesday, August 15, 2007 mother died from the indignities of Alzheimer's disease.

It has been a long, difficult, exhausting, and painful journey for everyone involved.

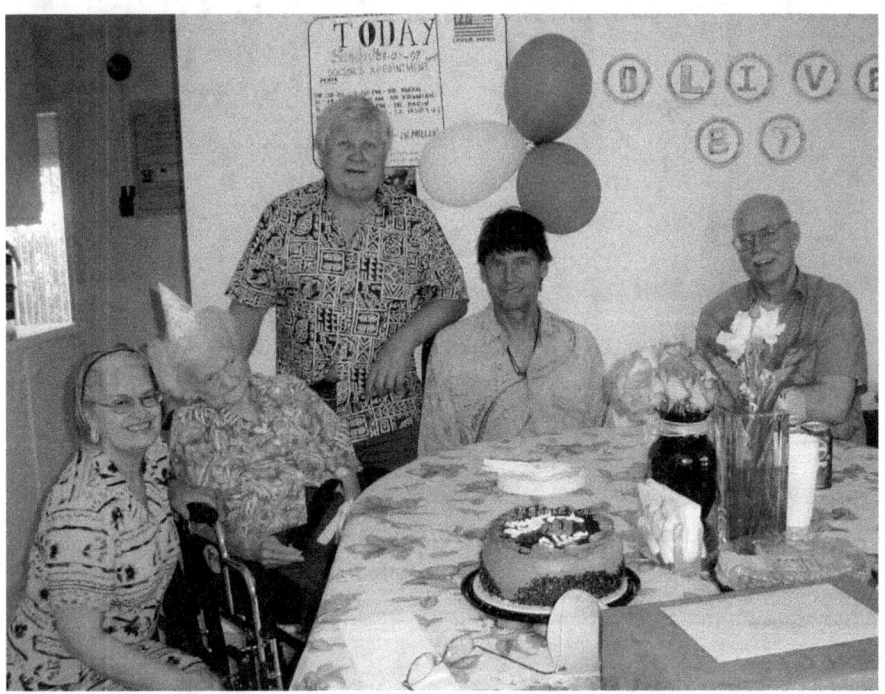

Figure 43: Olive on Her 87 Birthday, August 5, 2007

Stage 7: Very Severe Cognitive, Functional & Behavioral Decline/Severe Late-Stage Alzheimer's

The Final Days

During the first half of 2007, I spent the majority of my time dealing with cancer recovery, completing benefit forms for Olive's care, getting medications changed and insuring that mother remained on Hospice. In addition to thinking I was dying from cancer, I was also running out of money to pay for mother's care. During May 2007, my health improved and the pain in my shoulder and arms decreased.

In early July 2007 I received notification from Medicaid indicating Olive had been qualified to receive long-term care. During the middle of the July 2006, I received the billing information and details for beginning the benefits.

Immediately, Roger Eisele and I began meeting and inspecting nine local skilled nursing facilities in the area. Of the nine facilities, only one had an opening. The skilled nursing facility that had an opening had capacity to care for approximately 200 patients, was the newest, cleanest and seemed like a nice place to move mother from Leisure Living Board and Care. However, of the nine facilities, it was the one with the most deficiencies found in a recent California Department of Health inspection by nearly a factor of ten. Plus, whereas most skilled nursing facilities inspection reports were under ten pages, this skilled nursing facilities report was two-hundred-thirty-two pages long. The reality from our meetings and inspections is, when the government begins Medical Benefits, the government pays twice the cost of the care of a board and care and the quality of the care required by an Alzheimer's patient is cut in half. Benefits should support an Alzheimer patient's stay in a Board and Care Home where they usually receive more attention and avoid the move late in life that is likely to cause death.

The weekend before my mother passed away, I woke up early Sunday morning with my mind racing over alternatives and anguishing over the potential need of moving mother from Leisure Living to a skilled nursing facility due to almost completely running out of money. At the same time, my heart was beating rapidly as if I had walked up a steep incline. I got out of bed, drank a glass of milk, returned to bed and focused my mind on deep breathing and my breath until I fell back to sleep.

Later, the same day, August 5, John Madison, and Roger and Alice joined me to celebrate Olive's 87th birthday. A caregiver, Thelma, wheeled mother from her bedroom to the dining room where we were sitting. During the visit, Mother's head was tilted to the right, she was completely unresponsive and looked down at the floor during our entire ninety-minute visit. I cut a piece of cake for mother, but she would not open her mouth to eat the desert. On two previous visits the week before, mother had also been unresponsive. Up to this point, mother always smiled when I arrived or when she heard my voice. When I held her hand, I could feel her tighten her grip. But, for nearly the last month there was no response from mother during my visits.

The following week I contacted the attending Registered Hospice Nurse and voiced my concerns. On Friday, August 9, Kathy, the Hospice nurse who had evaluated mother the previous day called me. The following is the essence of our conversation from Kathy's observations that day:

- I mentioned to Kathy that mother was non-responsive each time I visited her during the last three weeks.
- Kathy said that Olive is calling out only when she is moved or during bathing, otherwise Olive is quiet.
- Her eyes are closed most of the time but open when she is being talked to.
- Cognitive abilities are declining.
- All physical vital signs (blood pressure, heart rate, body temperature, respiratory rate and weight) are stable.
- Skin is very pale.
- Muscle wasting is occurring.
- Bowls are working well.
- No skin breakdown.
- Olive is eating.

Stage 7: Very Severe Cognitive, Functional & Behavioral Decline/Severe Late-Stage Alzheimer's

- Caregivers have been advised to administer Ativan (Lorazepam)[63] for anxiety; Ativan instead Seroquel[64] and light morphine[65] dosage of .5 mg.
- Occasionally calling out, "Help me."
- Conversation ended at 10:52 (14 minutes total).

Summary: Kathy said, "I do not see anything that would cause me to believe Olive would not make it through the next thirty days."

On Saturday, August 11 and Sunday, August 12, mother developed a fever of 101 to 102 and her condition deteriorated significantly. Monday, Leisure Living attempted to contact me without success due to problems I was facing with my cell phone due to poor AT&T service in attempting to activate a new SIM card. Finally, I had to go to an independent cell phone service to resolve the problem. On Tuesday morning, August 14 I received a message from Buena Vista Hospice that mother's health was failing and I drove immediately to LLBC. Mother was lying in bed when I arrived. Her

---

[63] Lorazepam (also known by its brand name Ativan or Temesta) is a benzodiazepine drug with short to medium duration of action. It has all five intrinsic benzodiazepine effects: anxiolytic, sedative/hypnotic, anticonvulsant and muscle relaxant, to different extents. It is a powerful anxiolytic. It is a unique benzodiazepine insofar as it has also found use as an adjunct antiemetic in chemotherapy. Since its introduction in 1971, lorazepam's principal use has been in treating the symptom of anxiety. Among benzodiazepines, lorazepam has a relatively high addictive potential.

[64] Quetiapine (pronounced, kwe-TYE-a-peen), marketed by AstraZeneca as Seroquel and by Orion Pharma as Ketipinor, is an atypical antipsychotic used in the management of schizophrenia and bipolar I disorder, and off-label for a variety of other purposes.

[65] Morphine is a highly potent opiate analgesic drug and is the principal active agent in opium and the prototypical opioid. It is also a natural endocrine product in humans and other animals. Like other opioids, e.g., diacetylmorphine (heroin), morphine acts directly on the central nervous system (CNS) to relieve pain, and at synapses of the nucleus accumbens in particular. Studies done on the efficacy of various opioids have indicated that, in the management of severe pain, no other narcotic analgesic, other than Fentanyl (which has a higher potency, but is shorter acting), is more effective or superior to morphine[citation needed]. Morphine is highly addictive when compared to other substances; tolerance, physical and psychological dependences develop very rapidly.

eyes would open and close, but once again, mother was completely unresponsive. Later in the evening, I returned home for a restless night of sleep. The following is a summary of mother's last four days:

- Over the weekend, Mother started to develop a temperature that ranged from 101 to 102.
- Last food intake was on Monday, August 13.
- Vital signs went up and down with body metabolism.
- Heart Rate reached 154 bpm on Monday but was consistently around 100 bpm.
- Blood Pressure: 120/78 until Wednesday afternoon when blood pressure dropped and the RN could not get a reading.
- Respiratory Rate: normally 16-18, now 20; should be 14-20. It then dropped to twelve on Tuesday.
- Ice packs were placed around mother's arms, sides and neck to cool her down.
- Not responding to speech or sound.
- Classical music was played in the background (Bach and Beethoven).
- Only giving mother Atropine, to keep the air passages open and .5 mg of Morphine for comfort every four hours.
- All other medications were stopped.

Wednesday morning I returned to LL to be with Olive. The first thing I noticed was mother's apnea rate had changed. On Tuesday, mother would stop breathing for ten to twenty seconds and now the intervals were twenty to thirty seconds. In the early afternoon, the Certified Nursing Assistant (CNA) arrived and along with the two caregivers changed mother's bedding and gown. The CNA then took mother's temperature and it was 103.9. When the CNA could not get a blood pressure reading, she called the registered nurse (RN) at approximately two o'clock. The attending RN arrived quickly within five minutes, and was not able to get a reading from either arm or lower legs. She verified the temperature reading of 103.9 and they

Stage 7: Very Severe Cognitive, Functional & Behavioral Decline/Severe Late-Stage Alzheimer's

proceeded to place ice packs around mother's body. Next Jamie, the Hospice Chaplain, came by and spent a few moments with mother. Later, Paula, a Buena Vista Hospice Spiritual, Music Therapy and Dying Specialist, arrived. Sitting with Paula at the foot of mother's bed and with Paula's prompting, I reviewed mother's entire life. They say the last three things to go are hearing, lungs and heart. Assuming this is true, I am sure this was a very meaningful, pleasant and special time for mother. At 5:30 pm, Paula felt mother's arms, legs, and chest. She then turn to me and said, "Bob you have been a very good son the way you have cared for your mother, Olive is on her way, I must be going,." I walked out to the car with Paula and then walked approximately a quarter mile to the end of the street and back for some exercise. I then returned to mother's side. In that short period, I could visibly see Olive's circulation beginning to shut down. On her legs, I could see a mottling of the flesh. Similarly, mothers face as well as the area next to the arteries on the back of her neck, were sunken. At seven o'clock, Thelma came into the room and said, "Bob, come and eat, we have prepared some food for you." At the table was a single setting with two chicken thighs and some yams prepared Filipino style on a white plate. I sat alone at the table with sadness and ate the delicious food. The tasty food was exactly what my body needed. After eating, I returned to mother's room. Arlene brought in a bottle of water and I continued to sit by mother's side. At approximately 9:00 pm, I stood-up and felt mother's legs, arms, and her forehead. They were all stone cold. I placed my hand gently on her chest and could feel her lungs and heart working normally. Mothers eyes were only open slightly by approximately a quarter of an inch. Occasionally her eyes would open wide for a brief period of time. Tired, I returned to my home, spoke briefly with Ken Bayus and then lay down and slept for approximately ten minutes when Kathy called me. It was 10:45 pm and Kathy said, "Bob, your mother just peacefully passed away." I put my shoes on and drove immediately to Leisure Living. On the way, I cried and was very sad. However, by the time I arrived at leisure living I had regained my composure. Kathy, Thelma, Arlene and Nelson greeted me in the kitchen. Arlene gave me a hug and they all offered their condolences. I took a picture of them and then went into mother's bedroom. Olive was lying on her right side, in somewhat of a fetal position with her knees drawn up toward her chest. I looked down at mother who looked peaceful after all she had endured.

Kathy immediately called the USC Brain Research Study Group, which arrived in a little over an hour and quickly and efficiently removed mother's remains from LLB&C. Prior to the remains being removed, Kathy removed all of mother's jewelry and gave them to me. Before leaving LLB&C, I removed a collage of pictures from mother's wall (see Appendix J: Collage of Olive's Life, on page 292). Then I thanked the caregivers for being so caring, professional, thoughtful and kind during this very special time. I arrived home at approximately three o'clock and emailed a Notice of Death to mother's friends whose addresses I had previously entered into the computer.

The day after mother passed away, I received a call from a person at a skilled nursing facility informing me that they had an opening. I indicated we no longer had a need for a skilled nursing facility since mother passed away the night before.

This has been the most important, difficult, physically and emotionally draining sixty-eight month experience of my life. My heart has been heavy since mother's death. Dying of Alzheimer's disease is not for the faint hearted or a pretty sight at the end . . . the beauty is in the love you once shared!

Stage 7: Recommendation for Caregivers
Hospice

Hospice is a program designed to meet the special physical, psychological, social and spiritual needs of terminally ill patients who have six months or less to live. It is also designed to help support, educate and comfort the families of terminally ill patients.

Hospice provides skilled nursing, pain and symptom control, counseling and practical home care. An interdisciplinary team of professionals, who

Stage 7: Very Severe Cognitive, Functional & Behavioral Decline/Severe Late-Stage Alzheimer's

take a holistic approach to the patient's care, provides these services.

Hospice exists to provide support to and care for individuals with life-limiting conditions so they might live as fully and comfortably as possible. Emphasis is placed on the quality of life rather than on extending life by any means.

The concept of Hospice is broad. The purpose is to improve the quality of patient and/or family life by alleviating pain and recognizing that dying patients and their loved ones have special needs different from those whose treatment is designed to achieve a cure.

Hospice has grown from a volunteer movement to improve care for people dying alone, isolated, or in hospitals; to a significant part of the health care system. In 2005, more than 1.2 million individuals and their families received hospice care. Hospice is the only Medicare benefit that includes pharmaceuticals, medical equipment, twenty-four hour/seven day a week access to care and support for loved ones following a death. Most hospice care is delivered at home. Hospice care is also available to people in places like hospice residences, nursing homes, assisted living facilities, veterans' facilities, hospitals, and prisons.

Qualifying for Hospice Care is based on any patient with a life-limiting illness whose life expectancy is measured in months versus years.

Time Together

Time together during this phase will be spent exclusively at the place where the loved one resides. Keep your visit simple. You don't want to move and confuse the person. Communication can still take place even when the loved one can no longer speak. Focus on nonverbal communications; smile, rub the person's hands or body, play soothing music, bring enjoyable art for the person to view, an aromatic flower bouquet for the person to enjoy. Be careful not to over stimulate and confuse the loved one. They just enjoy your company at this point and know that someone who cares for them is by their side.

End of Life Arrangements

Autopsy, Mortuary, Order to Open the Grave Site, Church and Luncheon arrangements should all have been planned in advance. This is the last opportunity you will have to view the remains of the loved one and spend special time with the deceased. Reserve time to make this period memorable. If you are going to present a eulogy, rehearse giving it at the place where it is going to be presented if possible.

End of Life Events

Following Olive's death, her remains were taken to the University of Southern California, Brain Research Study Group where an autopsy was performed. On Saturday the remains were returned to the mortuary, the body was embalmed and placed in refrigerated storage awaiting shipment instructions for the funeral. Four days prior to the funeral, the remains were forwarded to the Funeral Home in Elkhorn, Wisconsin. The Saturday of Labor Day weekend the obituary which is illustrated in Appendix K: Olive's Obituary, beginning on page 293 appeared in local newspapers and the funeral was held the following Friday, September 7, 2007. During the service, Olive's son delivered a eulogy. The entire eulogy is in Appendix L: Olive's Eulogy, beginning on page 295. After the church service, a police escort led the funeral procession to the cemetery. As the hearse drove through town on the way to the cemetery, people along the street stopped what they were doing and paid their respect like people do in a small towns. All the vehicles in the incoming lane courteously pulled over and stopped. Internment was at Roselawn Cemetery, Lake Geneva, Wisconsin with a graveside service. Afterwards, friends and family members returned to a delicious luncheon at the First Evangelical Lutheran Church, Elkhorn, Wisconsin. This day left me with a lasting positive feeling from the people who came to pay their last respects to Olive's life. The day turned out the way mother would have wanted it to be.

Stage 7: Very Severe Cognitive, Functional & Behavioral Decline/Severe Late-Stage Alzheimer's

Grieving

A thoughtful e-mail from Ken Bayus a few days following mother's death provided me with comfort through this difficult time (see Appendix M: Ken Bayus Condolence eMail beginning on page 300).

Grief is a multi-faceted response to loss. Although conventionally focused on the emotional response to loss, it also has physical, cognitive, behavioral, social, and philosophical dimensions. Common to human experience is the death of a loved one, whether it is a friend, family member or another close companion, and in fact, the word "grief" comes from the same root as "grave." While the terms are often used interchangeably, bereavement often refers to the state of loss and grief to the reaction to loss.

Bereavement, while a normal part of life for us all, carries a degree of risk when limited support is available. Severe reactions to loss may carry over into familiar relations and cause trauma for children, spouses, other family members and friends, for example, there is an increased risk of marital breakup following the death of a child. Issues of personal faith and beliefs may also face challenges, as bereaved persons reassess personal definitions in the face of great pain. While many who grieve are able to work through their loss independently, accessing additional support from bereavement professionals may promote the process of healing. Grief counseling, professional support groups or educational classes and peer-led support groups are primary resources available to the bereaved. In the United States, local hospice agencies may be an important first contact for those seeking bereavement support.

Because of lack of time and energy following mother's death, scheduling the funeral and traveling back to Wisconsin, most of the potted plants on my patio also died in the late summer sun.

Grieving is a very personal experience.

Summary

Throughout this book, I have provided the reader with a textual description of Olive's decline from Alzheimer's disease. In this section, I will also provide you with a visual summary where you can clearly see Olive's health decline due to Alzheimer's.

I have often looked at the photo in Figure 44: Olive at her Home, August 1998 on page 157. This picture was taken while mother was experiencing double vision as a result of the concussion from her fall a couple of months earlier. This picture has bothered me for twenty years. Mother looks different in this photo than she did a few months earlier. In hindsight, to me mother was attempting to put on a healthy image, so as not worry anyone when in fact she was hurting physically and emotionally from the injury.

Figure 45 on page 158 is a photo summary of Olive which allows you to visually see her health decline with the progression of Alzheimer's disease. Figure 46 on page 159 through Figure 48 on page 161 include analysis comments with each photo.

Similarly, Figure 49 on page 162 is a photo summary of me. You can see in these pictures the health decline and aging affects as a result from the stress of caregiving. Personally, the experience has made me feel like I have aged twenty years. Figure 51 on page 163 and Figure 51 on page 164 includes brief background comments for each picture.

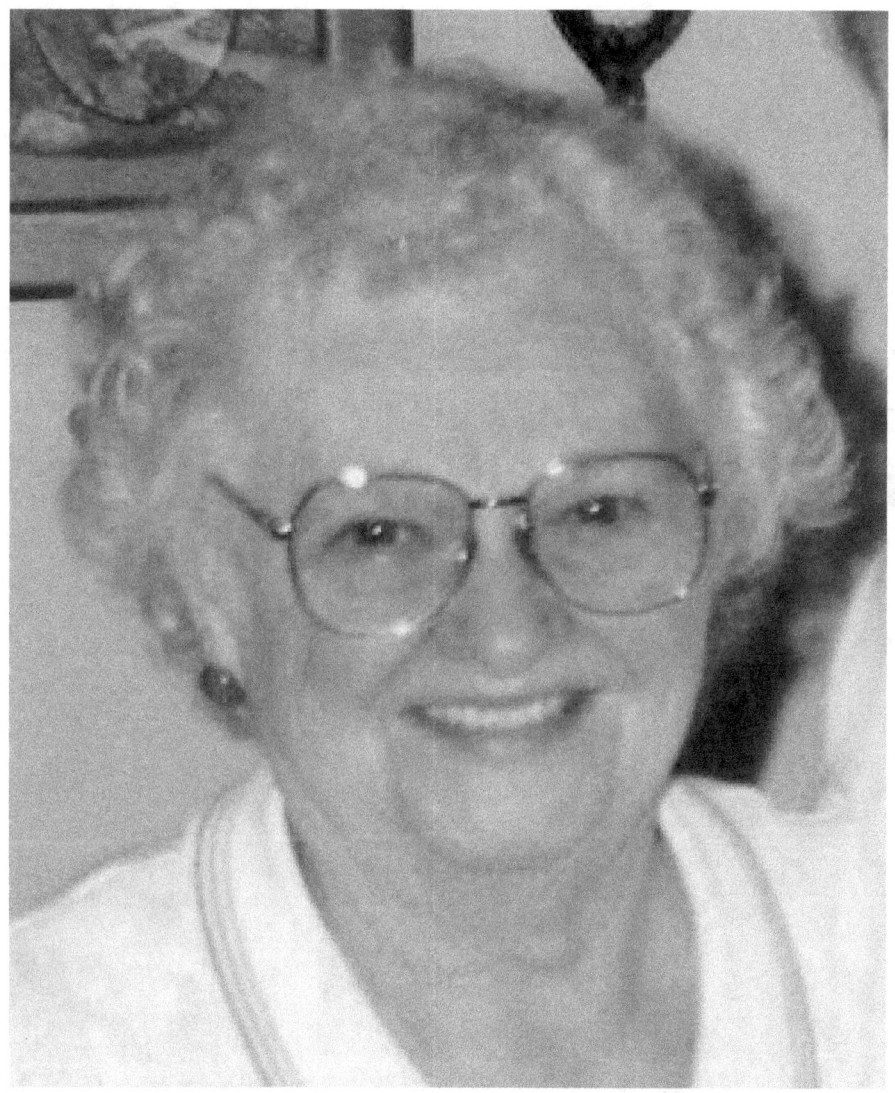

Figure 44: Olive at her Home, August 1998

Olive's Alzheimer's-Photo Summary

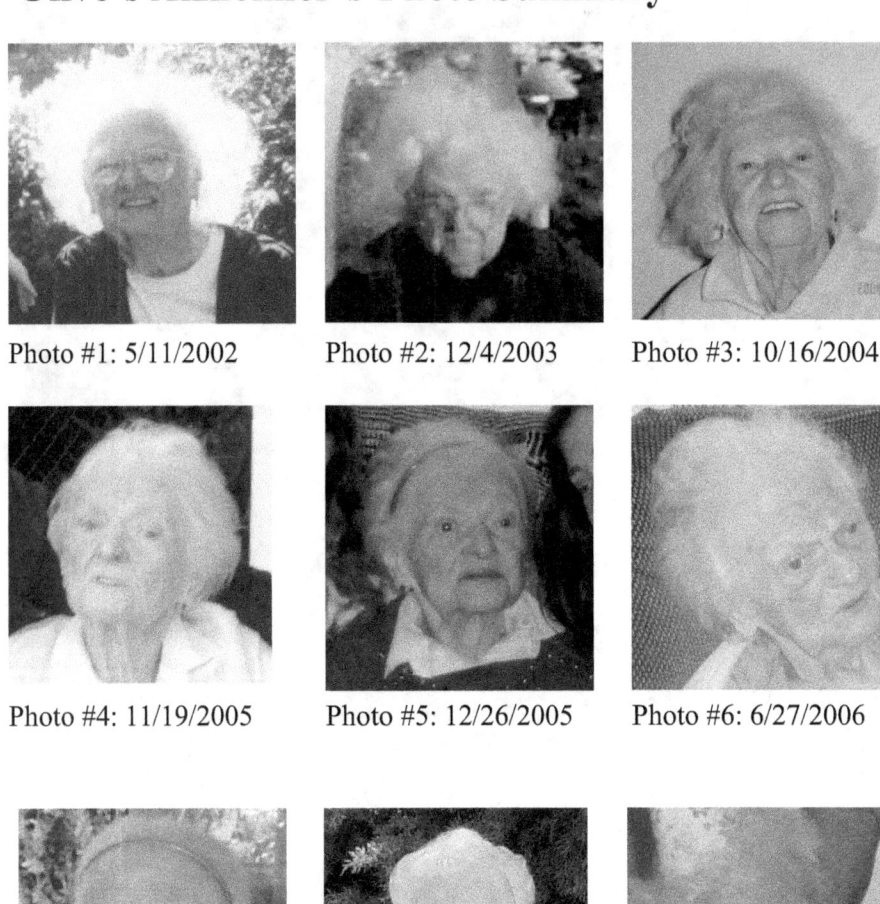

Photo #1: 5/11/2002   Photo #2: 12/4/2003   Photo #3: 10/16/2004

Photo #4: 11/19/2005   Photo #5: 12/26/2005   Photo #6: 6/27/2006

Photo #7: 8/5/2006   Photo #8: 6/2007   Photo #9: 8/5/2007

Figure 45: Photo Summary of Olive

Summary

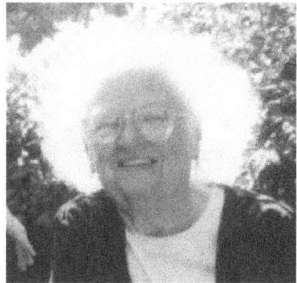 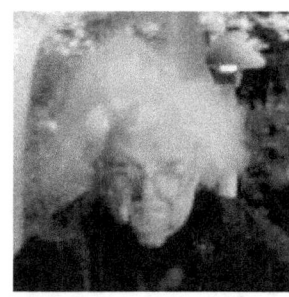 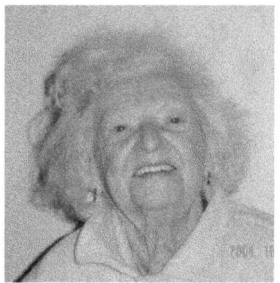

Photo #1: 5/11/2002
- This picture depicts Mother's typical happy ambience
- The way I will remember mother
- Excellent social skills
- Outgoing
- Talkative

Photo #2: 12/4/2003
- Becoming increasingly forgetful
- Experiencing difficulty walking
- Frustrated

Photo #3: 10/16/2004
- Happy
- Always positive
- Didn't want to concern anyone about her declining health
- Felt she would live to be nearly 100 like her mother

Figure 46: Photo Summary of Olive with Comments, 1 of 3

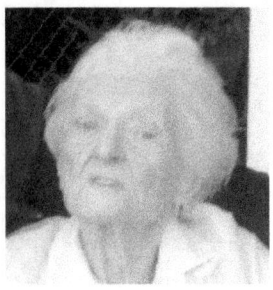 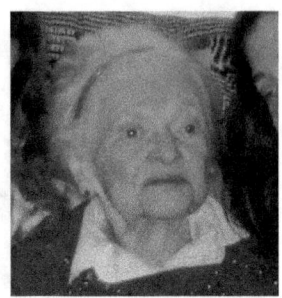 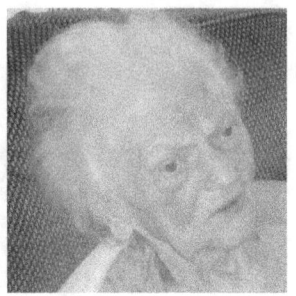

Photo #4: 11/19/2005

- Could not verbalize thoughts or ideas
- Stopped walking
- Only able to speak in short three or four word phrases

Photo #5: 12/26/2005

- Worried & terrified a good deal of the time.
- Lost 20 lbs
- Period of rapid health decline

Photo #6: 6/27/2006

- Frustrated
- Confused
- Angry
- Tearful

Figure 47: Photo Summary of Olive with Comments, 2 of 3

Summary

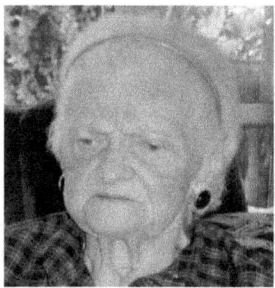

Photo #7: 8/5/2006
- Mother's 86 Birthday
- Sad because of her declining health
- Frustrated, but never violent

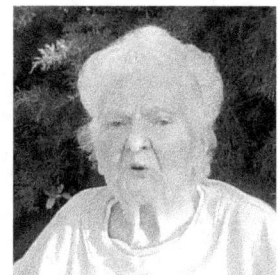

Photo #8: 6/2007
- At peace this day after I read from index cards about her wonderful life
- Gained back the weight she had lost.
- Unable to communicate verbally
- Attempted to speak but only able to make noises shortly after this photo was taken.

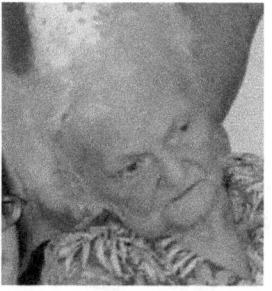

Photo #9: 8/5/2007
- Mother's 87 Birthday
- Uncommunicative
- Could not hold her head up
- Did not look at anyone
- Looked at the floor the entire visit
- No facial expression

Figure 48: Photo Summary of Olive with Comments, 1 of 3

Photo Summary of Caregiver, Bob

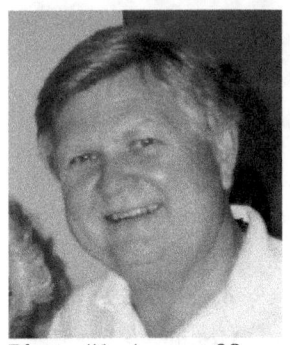
Photo #1: August 98

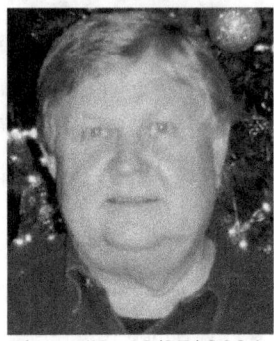
Photo #2: 12/27/ 2004

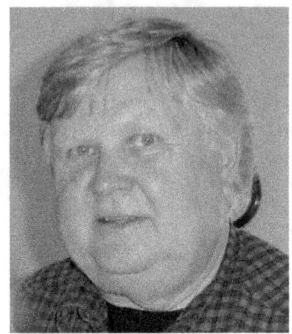
Photo #3: 5/19/2005

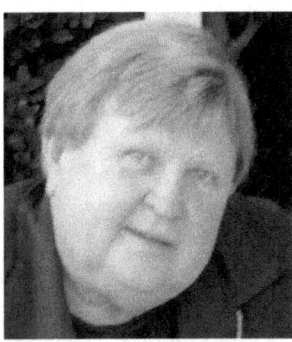
Photo #4: 11/19/ 2005

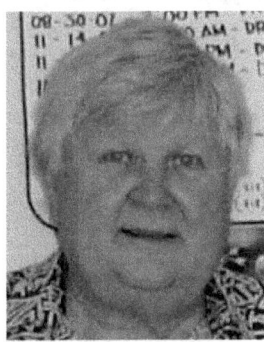
Photo #5: 8/5/2007

Figure 49: Photo Summary of Caregiver, Bob

Summary

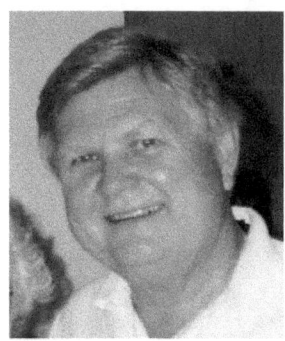

Photo #1: August 98
- Age 56
- Weight: 165 Lbs.
- Before Mother's Alzheimer's
- Very successful career period

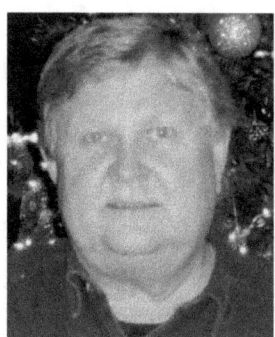

Photo #2: 12/27/ 2004
- Age 62
- Caregiving: 3-years

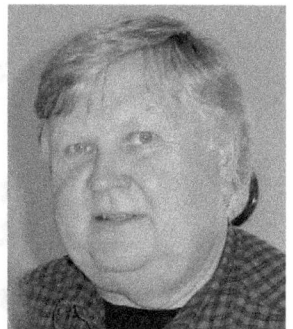

Photo #3: 5/19/2005
- Age 63
- Weight: 228 Lbs.
- Caregiving: 3-years and 5-months
- Very stressful time
- Health problems begin

Figure 50 Photo Summary of Caregiver with Comments, 1 of 2

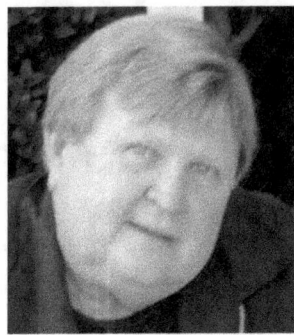 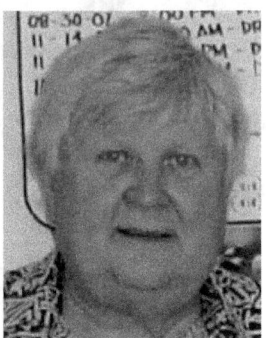

Photo #4: 11/19/ 2005	Photo #5: 8/5/2007

- Age 63
- Weight: 248 Lbs.
- Time of Caregiving: 3-years 11-months
- Very stressful, little energy, lots of pain
- Cancer diagnosed December 2005

- Age 65,
- Weight: 210 Lbs.
- Time of Caregiving: 5-years and 8-months
- 18-Months after cancer surgery
- Lost hair color, turned grey

Figure 51: Photo Summary of Caregiver with Comments, 2 of 2

Autopsy Results

Results, are described in Appendix I: Olive's Autopsy Results beginning on page 287. The autopsy was conducted by the Brain Research Study Group, Alzheimer's Disease Research Center, Memory and Aging Center, Keck School of Medicine, University of Southern California (USC). The USC Alzheimer's Disease Research Center is one of the thirty federally funded Alzheimer's Disease Centers (ADCs) across the country.

The report indicates, "The primary diagnosis was definite Alzheimer's disease based on mild cerebral atrophy and moderate to frequent amyloid deposition and neurofibrillary tangles. This report is consistent with the diagnosis from The Mayo Clinic conducted in early 2002. The secondary diagnosis was arteriolarsclerosis and atherosclerosis, which are the thickening of arterial walls and plaques in the blood vessels that interfere with circulation. The basilar vessels[66] were seventy-five percent occluded with atherosclerosis or plaque build-up."

The autopsy report specially confirms "definite Alzheimer's disease." Additionally, the report describes Vascular Dementia without specifically naming the disease. This was the first time that I was aware of a link between mother's heart disease and the Alzheimer's. Personally, I believe mother suffered from a combination of Alzheimer disease and Vascular Dementia.

I also personally believe this condition resulted initially from Rheumatic Fever as a teenager which resulted in lifelong heart problems or from the blood pressure and/or cardiac medications she took daily for over thirty years. It appears the disease started or worsened after the accident in 1998, when mother fell over, hit her head and was briefly in a coma. In summary, I

---

[66] In human anatomy, the basilar artery is one of the arteries that supply the brain with oxygen-rich blood. The two vertebral arteries and the basilar artery are sometimes together called the vertebrobasilar system, which supplies blood to the posterior part of circle of Willis and anastomoses with blood supplied to the anterior part of the circle of Willis from the carotid arteries.

believe mother died from a combination of Alzheimer's and vascular dementia.

The Cause of Death section, lists the cause of death as, "Alzheimer Dementia." The certificate inaccurately indicated Item 109, Biopsy Performed, No; Item 110, Autopsy Performed, No and Item 111, Used in Determining Cause, No. Items 109-111 should all be check, "Yes." These errors occurred since the Autopsy was performed after the Certificate of Death was completed and filed.

Cost of 68-Months Care

The cost of sixty eight months of caring for mother, not including lost income from being unable to work, amounted to in excess of a seven-hundred-fifty thousand dollars. Taking into account lost income, the overall cost exceeded a million dollars. Figure 1: Cost of Alzheimer's Care on page 19 and Figure 52: Table to Help Calculate Cost of Care on page 167 will help you calculate your own cost of care for a loved one.

Long Term Care Insurance

If a person chooses to take out a long term care insurance policy, they should pay particular attention to what the insurance covers. Many policies do not cover a facility such as a board and care or assisted living. Instead, many cover only nursing homes.

Long term care insurance is expensive. For example, if a policy is taken out at age fifty today, the insurance will cost approximately sixty-five dollars a month. When the cost of living adjustment is added into the benefits, the premium increases to close to two hundred dollars a month. Paying for long term care insurance with cost of living adjustments for approximately twenty to thirty years before it is needed is unaffordable for most families.

Instead, I believe a person's long term care insurance is found in family members and friends who the loved one has cultivated during their life.

SERVICE OR COST ITEM	DIRECT COST OF CARE	DIRECT COST PLUS LOST INCOME	COMMENT
Attending Physician			
Medication			
Living Costs			Food, Shelter, Clothing, etc.
Day Care at Senior Concerns			
Outside Caregiver			

Housing:
    Direct
    Utilities			

Board & Care			
Hospice			
Travel			
Lost Wages			
Total Cost			

Figure 52: Table to Help Calculate Cost of Care

National Crisis - Government Intervention Severely Needed

(Include letter to legislative representative explaining the Alzheimer's Crisis and need for government intervention.)

Life Turned Upside Down-Rebuilding a Caregiver's Shattered Dream

After the death of a loved one, the biggest challenge for caregiver(s) is restoring their life back to normal. Initially it is very hard to let go of this type of experience with a loved one. remember, life is only lived forward. The caregiving experience, unbeknown to the caregiver, has changed their life dramatically. The length of time a person has to deal with intense caregiving is usually four to eight years, although it can last as long as twenty or more years. It is normal during this time frame for the caregiver to withdraw from their career, friends and other activities. When the caregiving is over, the person may find it difficult to return to their previous career because of the absence or because they are older and no longer as valuable to an employer, plus the factor of age discrimination.

The caregiving experience is very intense and stressful with little support available outside the immediate family and support groups. Studies indicate that because of the intensity and stress of the experience, seventy percent of the caregivers either develop health problems or die before the person whose health they are managing. Afterward, it is common for the former caregiver to find their previous good health deteriorated from the stress. Previously, well planned hard work for retirement may now be compromised.

I hope this description of Olive's experience will provide the knowledge for effective care. May the book also open up more meaningful final days for the caregiver and their love one!

What You Can Do to Help in the Struggle Against Alzheimer Disease

At A Personal Level

At a personal level when AD is suspected, the most important action you can take is to educate yourself by reviewing the information in Appendix C: Diagnosing Alzheimer's, beginning on page 239 and seek diagnosis from one of the National Alzheimer's Research Centers listed in Appendix D:

Alzheimer Disease Research Centers, beginning on page 259. If the diagnosis is Alzheimer's disease, work quickly to assemble plans and insure all the proper legal documents are in order. You should have a three year plan which you update annually and monitor your own stress and health. A complete set of checklists and legal documents to assist you are described in Appendix A: Caregiver Essential Documents, beginning on page 181 and Appendix B: Legal Document Examples, beginning on page 199.

At A National Level

At a National Level the two most important actions you can take is to schedule an autopsy and insure that the Certificate of Death accurately states the cause of death as Alzheimer's disease. Results from the autopsy will go into a national database and be available to researchers seeking treatments and solutions for the disease. A death certificate indicating causes of death due to Alzheimer's will also help in increasing the funding level for the disease since funding in part is based on these statistics.

Lessons Learned

- Life today is extremely busy with careers, ambitions, commuting, family, home and autos. These things can deaden your awareness to what is really going on around you and what is important in life.
- Life is short, be aware of the mortality table, statistics on how people die and do not believe people are going to live forever.
- If you do not have your health, you truly do not have anything.
- Unfortunately, some people will attempt to take advantage of elderly people, especially when their health is declining. It is important for elderly people to have a trusted advocate to look after them and insure their financial and legal affairs are in order.
- Laws change regularly.
- Expect during your lifetime that you will have to take care of someone, just like someone is going to have to care for you.
- People used to feel that taking drugs might kill them. Now people take medications to stay alive.
- Set realistic goals for your life.
- Exercise daily, eat nutritious food and get adequate rest.
- Plan time to renew your body, mind and spirit.
- A person's world is limited only by their level of knowledge. Education is the only thing in life of which you cannot get too much. Commit to lifelong learning.
- Make each day count and celebrate life often.
- Other than your health, Love is really everything!

Conclusion

In this document I have described the key events with my mother's Alzheimer's disease. I have not mentioned a lot about the experience that the caregiver faces. It should be enough to be reminded that due to the stress brought on by caring for a person with Alzheimer's, half of the caregivers stop living or develop serious medical conditions before the loved one dies from the effects of Alzheimer's. This has been a long, agonizing sixty-eight months watching mother go from stubbornly insisting she could continue to live an independent life on her own to needing more and more care as a result of Alzheimer's disease and a series of strokes that took her mind and body. As Olive's only child, during this time I felt like I was on a forced march, trying to do my best but always feeling inadequate for the caregiving task.

During the early part of the last five years, mother and I got to know each other once again and had many good times and conversations during her stay in California. During this time mother saw The Chinese New Year's Parade in February 2002 and a Tony Bennett Concert at the Hollywood Bowl in August 2003. It took my good friend Jim Lindauer and I over two hours to transfer mother from the car to her theater seat for the Tony Bennett Concert. Olive also attended a Willie Nelson concert in November 2003 accompanied by her granddaughters, Aubrey and Shelby, friend, Ken Bayus, Ken's girlfriend and myself. Mother thoroughly enjoyed all these events. During the early summer of 2004, Olive began to decline rapidly. Alzheimer's is known as the designer's disease because a patient's condition continually changes. This is a terrifying experience for a person to face as they slowly but surely lose complete control of their mental faculties and associated physical capabilities. Alzheimer's is a terrible disease to handle. One day the person's condition seems to improve which gives you hope. The next day the condition worsens. Caregiving is very difficult, especially witnessing the constant decline of a loved one. First is the loss of short-term memory. Then as the disease progresses in the brain, it affects the muscular system and decreases mobility and increases frailness. It is like watching the slow disappearance of a person. The physical and emotional demands are very difficult for loved ones and caregivers to handle. To make things worse, since the cause of death of an Alzheimer's patient is usually listed as pneumonia, heart attack, stroke, etc., it has the least amount of research, prevention and treatment options of any major disease. Only four medications are currently available for treatment and all are very ineffective. To find a prevention or treatment for this dreadful disease, I urge everyone to support the National Alzheimer Association in any way they are able.

Summary

Midway through this journey, I was diagnosed with cancer at The Mayo Clinic and on Valentine's Day 2006 had surgery to remove the cancerous cells. A long recovery followed through April 2007. This made the journey even more difficult.

A couple of years ago, mother sat in a sun lit room at Leisure Living and as I approached, she turned to a caregiver and said proudly, "This is my son, Bob." Olive reached for my hand and looked at me intently, she was fully aware that her only child was by her side. I said to her as I did many times, "Mother, you have been a good mother, a wife, sister, sister-in law, grandmother and a good person. You have many wonderful friends. You have enjoyed a full, happy life." I continued to tell her, "I love you" and thanked her for everything she did for me.

The woman who nearly died giving me birth, nurtured me from infancy to adulthood, taught me how to read, count, pray, cross Elkhorn streets; whose belief in me provided the main motivation for major accomplishments in my life and protected me is no longer here. After being read the Lord's Prayer and the 23rd Psalm, Mother took a final deep breath and passed away peacefully on Wednesday evening, August 15, 2007 at 10:45 pm PST at age 87.

With mother's death, memories of the months of exhaustion, fear, self-doubt, second-guessing and, yes, complaining, "When will this ever end?" . . . instantly vanished. I had previously experienced the death of loved ones; my dad, grandmothers, aunts, uncles and friends, but never did it hurt like this. Even though I am in my middle sixties, I feel orphaned.

THIS HAS BEEN THE MOST DIFFICULT, PHYSICAL, EMOTIONALLY DRAINING, AND IMPORTANT EXPERIENCE OF MY LIFE!

There are experiences in life you cannot fully comprehend until you have intimately experienced them. The Alzheimer journey with mother has been this type of an experience. I am sure if Olive knew how much money was spent on her care or the concern I showed for her, it would have been enough to literally speaking, "kill her." In looking back at the effort, the most significant comment anyone has made of my efforts was by my friend Roger Eisele. Roger said, "I've been there, and I know. Some people go through their entire lives and never face a real trial. Some people face the test and cannot cut it. Others, though, face a terrible trial and do the necessary. Bob, a few days before your mother's death, when I saw you standing with your mother on her birthday and during all the years I have known you, you faced the test and you did what was necessary. You can be proud of that for the rest of your life." I know I did the right thing; I have no regrets for any of my care decisions for my mother.

Summary

When confusion ceases,
Tranquility comes,
when Tranquility comes,
Wisdom appears,
when Wisdom appears, Reality is seen.
                    Buddhist Saying

Reader Feedback Questionnaire

Please Provide Your Book Feedback

	ONE STAR	TWO STARS	THREE STARS	FOUR STARS	FIVE STARS
RATE THE BOOK:					
Overall Content Quality					
Organization					
Contents Support Goal Stated in Preface					
Research					
Writing					
Ease of Understanding					
Originality					
Alzheimer's Disease Education					
Caregiving Education					
Quality of Recommendations					
Value of Interior Images					
Value of Appendix					
Accuracy					
Overall Usefulness					
THE BOOK IS:					
Enlightening					
Touching					
Absorbing					
Informative					
BOOK IS GOOD FOR:					
Early Stage Alzheimer Patient					
Primary Caregiver					
Families & Friends of					

Reader Feedback Questionnaire

	ONE STAR	TWO STARS	THREE STARS	FOUR STARS	FIVE STARS
an Afflicted Love One with Alzheimer's Disease					
Professional Caregiver					
Public Libraries					
Primary Caregiver's Alzheimer's Reference					
Gift Giving					
Inspiration					
Intellectual Stimulation					
Understanding the Alzheimer's Crisis & Topical Conversation					

Three most useful headings

Three least useful headings

Reader Feedback Questionnaire

Three Recommendations for improvement

Reader Feedback Questionnaire

Thank you for taking the time to complete this questionnaire. Kindly, fold and mail the review to:

Robert Bublitz
4400 Sevenoaks
Westlake Village, CA 91361

Thank you for your review!

Appendix A: Caregiver Essential Documents

The following documents are included in this Appendix to help the organization of the Caregiver:

- Key Documents Summary
- Driver Reality Check
- Declining Memory Assessment
- Alzheimer's Patient Care Checklist
- Alzheimer Support Team
- Working Agenda for Caregiving Meetings
- Net Worth Calculation
- Monthly Income and Expense Budget
- Board & Care and Nursing Home Evaluation

Key Documents Summary

The following are key documents that should all be stored in one place and a copy should be made for the primary caregiver.

✓	DOCUMENT
	Personal Identification:
	Birth Certificate
	Marriage Certificate
	Divorce Documentation
	Certificate of Death for deceased spouse
	Social Security Card or at least a Social Security Card Number. A replacement should be ordered if the original cannot be found.
	Citizenship & naturalization paper's
	Passport and passport number
	Military Discharge Form DD-214. Required for any VA Disability
	Location of extra keys: home, garage, auto, boat, etc
	Safe Deposit Box location and keys
	Home Safe combination or keys
	Hidden Valuables
	Legal Documents:
	Trust or Will
	Durable Power of Attorney
	Health Care Directive
	Do Not Resuscitate Order (DNRO)
	Final Directive
	Medical Information:
	Medical Reports
	Patient Medical History
	List of Medications
	Insurance:
	Auto
	Home
	Medicare Supplement
	Medicare Part-D
	Long Term Care
	Financial Information

Appendix A: Essential Caregiver Information

✓	DOCUMENT
	Bank Accounts
	Credit Cards
	Pensions
	Social Security
	IRA
	Annuities
	401K Plans
	Military Retirement Benefits
	Military Disability Benefits
	Stocks & Bond Certificates
	Mutual Fund Account
	Royalties
	Partnership
	Debts & Loans (real estate, personal, credit union), etc.
	Real Estate Deeds
	Vehicle Title: Auto, boat, etc.
	Service records on auto, boat and major home appliances
	Easement & Right-of-Way Documents
	Businesses
	Items Stored or Loaned
	Rental Agreement
	Housing Contracts
	Name & phone number of real estate agents
	Business Agreements
	Cemetery Lot, Burial or Cremation policy
	Taxes: Copies of federal, state, local income and property tax returns for at least the last eight years

Driver Reality Check

When to Stop Driving[67]

We want to continue driving as long as we can do so safely. However, for many of us the time may come when we must limit or stop driving, either temporarily or permanently. The following advice may be able to assist you or someone you care about. What are the warning signs when someone should begin to limit driving or stop altogether?

Warning Signs

✓	ISSUE
	Feeling uncomfortable and nervous or fearful while driving
	Dents and scrapes on the car or on fences, mailboxes, garage doors, curbs etc.
	Difficulty staying in the lane of travel
	Getting lost
	Trouble paying attention to signals, road signs and pavement markings
	Slower response to unexpected situations
	Medical conditions or medications that may be affecting the ability to handle the car safely
	Frequent "close calls" (i.e. almost crashing)
	Trouble judging gaps in traffic at intersections and on highway entrance/exit ramps
	Other drivers honking at you and instances when you are angry at other drivers
	Friends or relatives not wanting to drive with you
	Difficulty seeing the sides of the road when looking straight ahead
	Easily distracted or having a hard time concentrating while driving
	Having a hard time turning around to check over your shoulder while backing up or changing lanes
	Frequent traffic tickets or "warnings" by traffic or law enforcement officers in the last year or two

---

[67] Adapted from, "When to Stop Driving,"
http://www.aarp.org/families/driver_safety/driver_safetyissues/a2004-06-21-whentostop.html

Appendix A: Essential Caregiver Information

If you notice one or more of these warning signs you may want to have your driving assessed by a professional or attend a driver refresher class (see resources at the bottom of this page). You may also want to consult with your doctor if you are having unusual concentration or memory problems, or other physical symptoms that may be affecting your ability to drive.

Adopting New Habits

✓	ISSUE
	Avoid Night Driving
	Avoid Rush Hour
	Avoid Freeways
	Avoid Driving in rain, strong winds, snow or other dangerous conditions
	Alternate Transportation
	Ride sharing
	Senior citizen transit pass
	Community vans
	Taxi
	Home delivery of groceries, prescriptions
	Shop via the Internet
	Ask friends, neighbors or volunteers

Declining Memory Assessment

TASK	COMPLETELY CAPABLE	SOME ASSISTANCE	NEEDS HELP
Dressing			
Grocery Shopping			
Preparing Meals			
Doing Laundry			
Home Cleaning			
Cutting Grass			
Shoveling Snow			
Personal Hygiene			
Transportation			
Paying Bills			
Taking Medications			
Remembering Medical, Dentist & Other Appointments			
Walking			

Appendix A: Essential Caregiver Information

Alzheimer's Patient Care Checklist

✓	ACTION	DATE DONE
	Enjoy as Much Personal Time Together with Your Afflicted Loved one as Possible	
	Diagnosis	
	Brain MRI/PET Scan	
	Discuss Wishes of Afflicted Love One	
	Discuss Impoverishment	
	Caregiver Plan to Build Physical & Emotional Endurance	
	May Want to Have a Professional Family Photo Taken	
	Primary Asset and Personal Property Inventory & Disposition Plan	
	Social Security Qualification for Disability Benefits	
	Medicaid Qualification for Long Term Care Benefits	
	Veterans Administration Qualification for Aid & Attendance Benefits for Widow of WWII Veteran	
	Select Doctor for house Call & Discuss Signing History of Certificates of Death for Past Alzheimer Patients	
	Research and Understand Drug which May be Necessary During Care	
	Will or Trust	
	Durable Power of Attorney	
	Health Care Directive	
	Do Not Resuscitate Order	
	Select Hospice Provider	
	Schedule Autopsy at an Alzheimer Research Center	
	Select Mortuary for Embalming or Cremation	
	Select Place for Final Service & Pall Bearers if Used	
	Select Monument	
	Select burial site	
	Final Arrangements	
	Early Stage Living Arrangement	
	Obtain a Free Annual Credit Reports (Experian,	

✓	ACTION	DATE DONE
	Equifax & Transunion & Fair Isaac Score	
	Long Term Living Arrangement	

Alzheimer Support Team

SPECIALTY	NAME	TELEPHONE	ADDRESS
Primary Caregiver			
Secondary Caregiver			
Immediate Family			
Close Friends			
Neighbors			
Emergency services: 911			
Family Doctor			
Ambulance			
Neurologist			
Pharmacist			
Cardiologist			
Oncologist			
Radiologist			
Pastor			
NAELA Attorney			
Social Worker			
Board & Care or Nursing Home			

Alzheimer's--What My Mother's Caregiving Taught Me

SPECIALTY	NAME	TELEPHONE	ADDRESS
Administrator			
Alzheimer Support Group friends			
Alzheimer Support Group Facilitator			
Certified Financial Planner			
CPA			
Dentist			
Home: Cleaning			
Home: Lawn Care			
Home: Snow Removal			
Hospice, Dying /Spiritualist Specialist			
Hospice, GM			
Hospice, Pastor			
Hospice, RN			
Hospice: CNA			
Hospice, Social Worker			
Insurance Co. Medicare Supplement			
Insurance Co.: Auto			
Insurance Co.: Household			
Insurance Co.: Life			
Insurance Co.: Part-D			

Appendix A: Essential Caregiver Information

SPECIALTY	NAME	TELEPHONE	ADDRESS
Stock Broker			
Other			

Agenda for Caregiving Meetings

Ground Rules:

- Include everyone who cares for the welfare of the loved one as well as the loved one who needs the care. Also, include family members and close friends.
- Agree to respect one another's view on those subjects where there is disagreement. Building consensus means being willing to meet in the middle. Everyone sees things differently and everyone's story is valid.
- Do not digress into the past. Agree at the beginning that this meeting is not the place to bring up "old feeling and emotions." Focus on the needs of the loved one whose care is the topic to be discussed.
- Share the load of caregiving. No one should be afraid to ask for help. It is important to volunteer and ask, "How can I help?"

ISSUES TO BE DISCUSSED		
Task	Person Responsible	Due Date or Frequency
Follow-up Steps (e-Mail, Telephone, Circulate Copies, Mail, etc.		

Net Worth Calculation Worksheet

	HUSBAND	WIFE	COMBINED
Asset:			
Annuities			
Bonds			
Business			
Cash			
Checking Accounts			
Insurance Policies: Paid-Up			
IRAs/Keoghs			
Mutual Funds			
Personal Property			
Real Estate: Home			
Real Estate: Other			
Stocks			
Vehicles: Auto			
Vehicles: Other			
Total Assets			
Liabilities:			
Credit Card Debt			
Loan: Auto			
Loan: Mortgage			
Loans: Other			
Other Liabilities			
Taxes: Unpaid			
Total Liabilities			
Total Assets from Above less Total Liabilities = NET WORTH			

Monthly Income and Expense Budget Worksheet

	MONTH	COMMENT
Expenses:		
Auto: Fuel		
Auto: Insurance		
Auto: Loan		
Auto: Maintenance		
Care: Dental		
Clothing		
Credit Cards		
Entertainment		
Fees: Financial		
Fees: Legal		
Food		
Gifts		
Home Cleaning		
Home Maintenance		
Home: Insurance		
Insurance: Life		
Insurance: Long Term Care		
Insurance: Medicare Supplement		
Insurance: Medicare: Part D		
Medical Care		
Mortgage/Rent		
Personal Care		
Pets		
Postage		
Taxes: Federal		
Taxes: Other		
Taxes: State		
Utilities: Gas		
Utilities: Internet		
Utilities: Telephone		
Utilities: Cable		

Appendix A: Essential Caregiver Information

	MONTH	COMMENT
Utilities: Electric		
Utilities: Trash Collection		
Utilities: Water		
Total Expenses		
Income:		
Husband		
Wife		
Combined Income		
Annuity		
Business		
Dividends		
Interest		
IRA/Keogh		
Pension		
Rental		
Social Security		
Trust		
Veterans Benefits		
Wages		
Other		
Total Income		
Less Total Expenses		
Net Income		
Notes		

Board & Care/Nursing Home Evaluation[68]

FACILITY NAME:							
Administrator							
Address:							
City:							
Phone:							
Check		First Visit		Second Visit		Dates	
		Morning		Afternoon		Evening	
Circle	Mon	Tue	Wed	Thu	Fir	Sat	Sun
Care Issues						Yes	No
Does the facility have a fresh smell?							
Are residents clean and well groomed?							
Do staff members interact well with residents?							
Are residents participating in activities and exercise?							
Do the residents have the same caregiver on a regular basis?							
Does the staff respond quickly to calls for help?							
Is fresh water available in the room?							
Does the food look and smell fresh and taste good?							
Are residents offered choices of food at meal times?							
Are residents who need assistance eating or drinking receiving it?							
Are there nutritious snacks available throughout the day and evening?							
Is physical therapy available for as long as the resident needs it?							
Does the staff have special training to deal with Alzheimer's and other dementia?							
Are there special services for special Alzheimer's needs?							
Quality of Life							
Does the staff knock before entering a resident's room?							
Are the doors shut when a resident is being dressed or bathed?							
Is the facility an easy place for family and friends to visit?							

[68] Adapted from "Caring for your Parents - The Complete Family Guide," Hugh Delehanty & Ellinor Ginler, AARP/Sterling, 2005, ISBN 13:978-1-4027-5857-7

Appendix A: Essential Caregiver Information

Does the facility meet cultural, religious and language needs?		
Are there outdoor areas and help for residents who wish to use them?		
Are the residents allowed to make choices about daily routine such as bedtime, when to bathe or when to eat?		
Are the residents allowed to have personal articles of furniture and mementoes in their rooms?		
Is the staff friendly, considerate and helpful?		
Does the facility have a friendly, homelike ambience?		
Safety		
Are rooms, stairs and hallways well lighted?		
Are exits marked?		
Do the hallways have handrails?		
Do the rooms, bathrooms and showers have grab bars and call buttons?		
Are there safety locks on the doors and windows?		
Are there security and fire safety systems?		
Is there an emergency generator or alternative power source?		
Is the floor plan logical and easy to follow?		
Does the room have its own bathroom and shower?		
General		
Is the facility Medicaid certified?		
Has the license ever been revoked?		
Is the facility accepting new patients?		
Is there a waiting period for admission?		
Does the facility conduct background checks on all of the staff?		
How many licensed registered nurses (RNs) are on duty during each shift?		
What is the patient to staff ratio?		
What is the RN [registered nurse]/patient ratio?		
What is the RN, LPN, CNA (certified nurses aide)/patient ratios?		
Does the nursing home have an active family council?		
What is the visiting policy?		
Are care planning meetings held at times convenient for family members to attend?		

How many discrepancies did the facility receive on the last state inspection? When was the last state inspection?		

Appendix B: Legal Document Examples

The following documents, which are included in this Appendix, are examples of legal documents you may generate on your home computer from a variety of software companies. The examples in this book use an older version of WillMaker Software:[69]

- Will: Example from the State of New York
- Living Basic Trust: Example from the State of California
- General Power of Attorney: Example from the State of Texas
- Health Care Directive: Example from the State of Minnesota. This document also includes instruction that come with each type of document from Quicken.
- Final Arrangements: Example from the State of Florida

Note, for your own personal use, an up to date version of software should be used to reflect the current laws in the appropriate state.

Most of these software packages come with instruction for recording and filing the document. Additionally they come with references for other sources of help. Additionally, I have included the following actual documents used in Olive's Care to provide you with examples:

- Do Not Resuscitate Orders (DNRO)
- Doctor's Order for Hospice Care

Quicken WillMaker Doesn't Provide Legal Advice

Nolo, provider of legal content for Quicken WillMaker, publishes legal forms that are useful in many situations. But we can't tell you whether or not a form is right for you, given your circumstances. If you want advice geared

---

[69] Nolo developed WillMaker which is marketed by Quicken. The product is available from either nolo.com, quicken.intuit.com or other resellers.

to your specific situation, consult an expert. No general legal form is a substitute for personalized advice from a knowledgeable lawyer licensed to practice law in your state.

Quicken WillMaker Plus 2005 version 4.0

Health Care Directive version 4.0.0.0

Copyright 2004 by Nolo

Will-An Example in the State of New York

Will of John Doe

Part 1. Personal Information

I, John Doe, a resident of the State of New York, West-Chester County, declare that this is my will. My Social Security number is 123-45-6789.

Part 2. Revocation of Previous Wills

I revoke all wills and codicils that I have previously made.

Part 3. Marital Status

I am married to Mary Doe.

Part 4. Children

I have the following children now living: Bob Doe and Kathy Doe.

Part 5. Grandchildren

I have the following grandchild now living: Holly Doe.

Part 6. Disposition of Property

All beneficiaries must survive me for 45 days to receive property under this will. As used in this will, the phrase "survive me" means to be alive or in existence as an organization on the 45th day after my death.

All personal and real property that I leave in this will shall pass subject to any encumbrances or liens placed on the property as security for the repayment of a loan or debt.

If I leave property to be shared by two or more beneficiaries, it shall be shared equally by them unless this will provides otherwise.

If I leave property to be shared by two or more beneficiaries, and any of them does not survive me, I leave his or her share to the others equally unless this will provides otherwise for that share.

"Entire estate" means all property I own at my death that is subject to this will.

I leave my entire estate to my wife Mary Doe. If my wife Mary Doe does not survive me, I leave my entire estate to my children Bob Doe and Kathy Doe in equal shares.

If Mary Doe, Bob Doe and Kathy Doe all do not survive me, I leave my entire estate to Holly Doe.

Part 7. Executors

I name Bob Doe and Kathy Doe to serve together as my joint executors.

If Bob Doe or Kathy Doe is unwilling or unable to serve as executor, the other executor shall continue to serve.

No executor shall be required to post bond.

Part 8. Executor's Powers

I direct my executor to take all actions legally permissible to have the probate of my will done as simply and as free of court supervision as possible under the laws of the state having jurisdiction over this will, including filing a petition in the appropriate court for the independent administration of my estate.

I grant to my executor the following powers, to be exercised as he or she deems to be in the best interests of my estate:

1) To retain property without liability for loss or depreciation.

2) To dispose of property by public or private sale, or exchange, or otherwise, and receive and administer the proceeds as a part of my estate.

3) To vote stock, to exercise any option or privilege to convert bonds, notes, stocks or other securities belonging to my estate into other bonds, notes, stocks or other securities, and to exercise all other rights and privileges of a person owning similar property.

4) To lease any real property in my estate.

5) To abandon, adjust, arbitrate, compromise, sue on or defend and otherwise deal with and settle claims in favor of or against my estate.

6) To continue or participate in any business which is a part of my estate, and to incorporate, dissolve or otherwise change the form of organization of the business.

The powers, authority and discretion I grant to my executor are intended to be in addition to the powers, authority and discretion vested in him or her by operation of law by virtue of his or her office, and may be exercised as often as is deemed necessary or advisable, without application to or approval by any court.

Part 9. Payment of Debts

Except for liens and encumbrances placed on property as security for the repayment of a loan or debt, I want all debts and expenses owed by my estate to be paid in the manner provided for by the laws of New York.

Part 10. Payment of Taxes

I want all estate and inheritance taxes assessed against property in my estate or against my beneficiaries to be paid using the following assets, in the order listed: My Savings Account with Nations Bank.

Part 11. No Contest Provision

If any beneficiary under this will contests this will or any of its provisions, any share or interest in my estate given to the contesting beneficiary under this will is revoked and shall be disposed of as if that contesting beneficiary had not survived me.

Part 12. Severability

If any provision of this will is held invalid, that shall not affect other provisions that can be given effect without the invalid provision.

Signature

I, John Doe, the testator, sign my name to this instrument, this

_____ day of _____, _____, at

_____. I declare that I sign and

execute this instrument as my last will, that I sign it willingly, and that I execute it as my free and voluntary act. I declare that I am of the age of majority or otherwise legally empowered to make a will, and under no constraint or undue influence.

Signature: _____

Witnesses

We, the witnesses, sign our names to this instrument, and declare that the testator willingly signed and executed this instrument as the testator's last will.

In the presence of the testator, and in the presence of each other, we sign this will as witnesses to the testator's signing.

To the best of our knowledge, the testator is of the age of majority or otherwise legally empowered to make a will, is mentally competent and under no constraint or undue influence.

We declare under penalty of perjury that the foregoing is true and correct, this _____ day of _____, _____, at

_____.

Witness #1: _____

Residing at: _____

Witness #2: _____

Residing at: _____

Living Basic Trust-An Example in the State of California

Declaration of Trust

Part 1. Trust Name

This revocable living trust shall be known as the John Doe Revocable Living Trust.

Part 2. Declaration of Trust

John Doe, called the grantor, declares that he has transferred and delivered to the trustee all his interest in the property described in Schedule A attached to this Declaration of Trust. All of that property is called the "trust property." The trustee hereby acknowledges receipt of the trust property and agrees to hold the trust property in trust, according to this Declaration of Trust.

The grantor may add property to the trust.

Part 3. Terminology

The term "this Declaration of Trust" includes any provisions added by valid amendment.

Part 4. Amendment and Revocation

A. Amendment or Revocation by Grantor

The grantor may amend or revoke this trust at any time, without notifying any beneficiary. An amendment must be made in writing and signed by the grantor. Revocation may be in writing or any manner allowed by law.

B. Amendment or Revocation by Other Person

The power to revoke or amend this trust is personal to the grantor. A conservator, guardian or other person shall not exercise it on behalf of the grantor, unless the grantor specifically grants a power to revoke or amend this trust in a Durable Power of Attorney.

Part 5. Payments From Trust During Grantor's Lifetime

The trustee shall pay to or use for the benefit of the grantor as much of the net income and principal of the trust property as the grantor requests. Income shall be paid to the grantor at least annually. Income accruing in or paid to trust accounts shall be deemed to have been paid to the grantor.

Part 6. Trustees

A. Trustee
John Doe shall be the trustee of this trust.

B. Trustee's Responsibilities
The trustee in office shall serve as trustee of all trusts created under this Declaration of Trust, including children's subtrusts.

C. Terminology
In this Declaration of Trust, the term "trustee" includes successor trustees or alternate successor trustees serving as trustee of this trust. The singular "trustee" also includes the plural.

D. Successor Trustee
Upon the death or incapacity of John Doe, the trustee of this trust and of any children's subtrusts created by it shall be Kathy Doe, Bob Doe and Mary Doe. All of the successor trustees must consent, in writing, to any transaction involving the trust or trust property.

E. Resignation of Trustee
Any trustee in office may resign at any time by signing a notice of resignation. The resignation shall be delivered to the person or institution who is either named in this Declaration of Trust, or appointed by the trustee under Section F of this Part, to next serve as the trustee.

F. Power to Appoint Successor Trustee
If no one named in this Declaration of Trust as a successor trustee or alternate successor trustee is willing or able to serve as trustee, the last acting trustee may appoint a successor trustee and may require the posting of a reasonable bond, to be paid for from the trust property. The appointment must be made in writing, signed by the trustee and notarized.

G. Bond
No bond shall be required for any trustee named in this Declaration of Trust.

H. Compensation
No trustee shall receive any compensation for serving as trustee, unless the trustee serves as a trustee of a child's subtrust created by this Declaration of Trust.

I. Liability of Trustee
With respect to the exercise or non-exercise of discretionary powers granted by this Declaration of Trust, the trustee shall not be liable for

actions taken in good faith. Such actions shall be binding on all persons interested in the trust property.

Part 7. Trustee's Management Powers and Duties

A. Powers Under State Law

The trustee shall have all authority and powers allowed or conferred on a trustee under California law, subject to the trustee's fiduciary duty to the grantors and the beneficiaries.

B. Specified Powers

The trustee's powers include, but are not limited to:

1. The power to sell trust property, and to borrow money and to encumber trust property, including trust real estate, by mortgage, deed of trust or other method.

2. The power to manage trust real estate as if the trustee were the absolute owner of it, including the power to lease (even if the lease term may extend beyond the period of any trust) or grant options to lease the property, to make repairs or alterations and to insure against loss.

3. The power to sell or grant options for the sale or exchange of any trust property, including stocks, bonds, debentures and any other form of security or security account, at public or private sale for cash or on credit.

4. The power to invest trust property in every kind of property and every kind of investment, including but not limited to bonds, debentures, notes, mortgages, stock options, futures and stocks, and including buying on margin.

5. The power to receive additional property from any source and add it to any trust created by this Declaration of Trust.

6. The power to employ and pay reasonable fees to accountants, lawyers or investment experts for information or advice relating to the trust.

7. The power to deposit and hold trust funds in both interest-bearing

and non-interest bearing accounts.

8. The power to deposit funds in bank or other accounts, whether or not they are insured by the FDIC.

9. The power to enter into electronic fund transfers or safe deposit arrangements with financial institutions.

10. The power to continue any business of the grantor.

11. The power to institute or defend legal actions concerning this trust or the grantor's affairs.

12. The power to execute any documents necessary to administer any trust created by this Declaration of Trust.

13. The power to diversify investments, including authority to decide that some or all of the trust property need not produce income.

Part 8. Incapacity of Grantor

If the grantor becomes physically or mentally incapacitated, whether or not a court has declared the grantor incompetent or in need of a conservator or guardian, the successor trustee named in Part 6 shall be trustee. Incapacity must be certified in writing by a licensed physician.

In that event, the trustee shall manage the trust property. The trustee shall use any amount of trust income or trust property necessary for the grantor's proper health care, support, maintenance, comfort and welfare, in accordance with the grantor's accustomed manner of living. Any income not spent for the benefit of the grantor shall be accumulated and added to the trust property. Income shall be paid to the grantor at least annually. Income accruing in or paid to trust accounts shall be deemed to have been paid to the grantor.

The successor trustee shall manage the trust until a licensed physician certifies in writing that the grantor is again able to manage his affairs.

Part 9. Death of a Grantor

When the grantor dies, this trust shall become irrevocable. It may not be amended or altered except as provided for by this Declaration of Trust. It may be terminated only by the distributions authorized by this Declaration of Trust.

The trustee may pay out of trust property such amounts as necessary for payment of the grantor's debts, estate taxes and expenses of the grantor's last illness and funeral.

Part 10. Beneficiaries

At the death of the grantor, the trustee shall distribute the trust property as follows:

> 1. Mary Doe, Kathy Doe and Bob Doe shall be given John Doe's interest in the trust property as follows:

> Mary Doe shall receive a 1/2 share.

> Kathy Doe shall receive a 1/4 share.

> Bob Doe shall receive a 1/4 share.

> 2. Holly Doe shall be given all John Doe's interest in the trust property not otherwise specifically and validly disposed of by this Part.

All distributions are subject to any provision in this Declaration of Trust that creates a child's subtrust or a custodianship under the Uniform Transfers to Minors Act.

A beneficiary must survive the grantor for 120 hours to receive property under this Declaration of Trust. As used in this Declaration of Trust, to survive means to be alive or in existence as an organization.

All personal and real property left through this trust shall pass subject to any encumbrances or liens placed on the property as security for the repayment of a loan or debt.

If property is left to two or more beneficiaries to share, they shall share it equally unless this Declaration of Trust provides otherwise. If any of them does not survive the grantor, the others shall take that beneficiary's share, to share equally, unless this Declaration of Trust provides otherwise.

Part 11. Grantor's Right to Homestead Tax Exemption

If the grantor's principal residence is held in trust, grantor has the right to possess and occupy it for life, rent-free and without charge except for taxes, insurance, maintenance and related costs and expenses. This right is intended to give grantor a beneficial interest in the property and to ensure that grantor does not lose eligibility for a state homestead tax exemption for which he otherwise qualifies.

Part 12. Severability of Clauses

If any provision of this Declaration of Trust is ruled unenforceable, the remaining provisions shall stay in effect.

Certification of Grantor

I certify that I have read this Declaration of Trust and that it correctly states the terms and conditions under which the trust property is to be held, managed and disposed of by the trustee, and I approve the Declaration of Trust.

_____   Dated: _____
John Doe, Grantor and Trustee

CERTIFICATE OF ACKNOWLEDGMENT OF NOTARY PUBLIC

State of California   )

) ss.

County of _____)

On _____, _____ before me,

_____, a notary public in and for said state, personally appeared John Doe, personally known to me (or proved on the basis of satisfactory evidence) to be the person whose name is subscribed to the within instrument, and acknowledged to me that he executed the same in his authorized capacity, and that by his signature on the instrument the person, or the entity upon behalf of which the person acted, executed the instrument.

         WITNESS my hand and official seal.

        _____

        Notary Public for the State of Calif.

[NOTARIAL SEAL]   My commission expires: _____

SCHEDULE A

1. Home at 3400 Paradise Lane.

Durable Power of Attorney for Financial Management- An Example in the State of Texas

1. Principal and Attorney-in-Fact

PRINCIPAL

John Doe

2300 Paradise Lane

Paradise Valley, Texas 75201

I, John Doe, appoint the persons named below as my attorneys-in-fact to act for me in any lawful way with respect to the powers delegated in Part 5 below.

ATTORNEYS-IN-FACT

Mary Doe

200 At Last Acres

Paradise Valley, Minnesota 55901 U.S.A.

Day phone: 300-572-9132

Evening phone: 300-672-9173

Bob Doe

233 Valley Drive

Paradise Valley, California 03000 U.S.A.

Day phone: 300-256-9243

Evening phone: 300256-3819

Kathy Doe

4362 S.E. 18th

Mountain High, California 55901

2. Authorization of Attorneys-in-Fact

My attorneys-in-fact must act jointly.

3. Delegation of Authority

My attorney-in-fact may delegate, in writing, any authority granted under this durable power of attorney to a person he or she selects. Any such delegation shall state the period during which it is valid and specify the extent of the delegation.

4. Effective Date

This power of attorney is effective immediately, and shall continue in effect if I become incapacitated or disabled.

5. Powers of Attorney-in-Fact

I grant my attorney-in-fact power to act on my behalf in the following matters, as indicated by my initials next to each granted power.

INITIALS

X_____	(1) Real estate transactions.
X_____	(2) Tangible personal property transactions.
X_____	(3) Stock and bond, commodity, option and other securities transactions.
X_____	(4) Banking and other financial institution transactions.
X_____	(5) Business operating transactions.
X_____	(6) Insurance and annuity transactions.
X_____	(7) Estate, trust, and other beneficiary transactions.
X_____	(8) Living trust transactions.
X_____	(9) Legal actions.
X_____	(10) Personal and family care.
X_____	(11) Government benefits.
X_____	(12) Retirement plan transactions.
X_____	(13) Tax matters.

These powers are defined in Part 12, below.

6. Compensation and Reimbursement of Attorney-in-Fact

My attorney-in-fact shall not be compensated for services, but shall be entitled to reimbursement, from my assets, for reasonable expenses. Reasonable expenses include but are not limited to reasonable fees for information or advice from accountants, lawyers or investment experts relating to my attorney-in-fact's responsibilities under this power of attorney.

7. Personal Benefit to Attorney-in-Fact

My attorney-in-fact may buy any assets of mine or engage in any transaction he or she deems in good faith to be in my interest, no matter what the interest or benefit to my attorney-in-fact.

8. Commingling by Attorney-in-Fact

My attorney-in-fact may commingle any of my funds with any funds of his or hers.

9. Liability of Attorney-in-Fact

My attorney-in-fact shall not incur any liability to me, my estate, my heirs, successors or assigns for acting or refraining from acting under this document, except for willful misconduct or gross negligence. My attorney-in-fact is not required to make my assets produce income, increase the value of my estate, diversify my investments or enter into transactions authorized by this document, as long as my attorney-in-fact believes his or her actions are in my best interests or in the interests of my estate and of those interested in my estate. A successor attorney-in-fact shall not be liable for acts of a prior attorney-in-fact.

10. Reliance on This Power of Attorney

Any third party who receives a copy of this document may rely on and act under it. Revocation of the power of attorney is not effective as to a third party until the third party has actual knowledge of the revocation. I agree to indemnify the third party for any claims that arise against the third party because of reliance on this power of attorney.

11. Severability

If any provision of this document is ruled unenforceable, the remaining provisions shall stay in effect.

12. Definition of Powers Granted to Attorney-in-Fact

The powers granted in Part 5 above authorize my attorney-in-fact to do the following:

(1) Real estate transactions

My attorney-in-fact may act for me in any manner to deal with all or any part of any interest in real property that I own at the time of execution of this document or later acquire, under such terms, conditions and covenants as my attorney-in-fact deems proper. My attorney-in-fact's powers include but are not limited to the power to:

(a) Accept as a gift, or as security for a loan, reject, demand, buy, lease, receive or otherwise acquire ownership of possession of any estate or interest in real property.

(b) Sell, exchange, convey with or without covenants, quitclaim, release, surrender, mortgage, encumber, partition or consent to the partitioning of, grant options concerning, lease, sublet or otherwise dispose of any interest in real property.

(c) Maintain, repair, improve, insure, rent, lease, and pay or contest taxes or assessments on any estate or interest in real property I own or claim to own.

(d) Prosecute, defend, intervene in, submit to arbitration, settle and propose or accept a compromise with respect to any claim in favor of or against me based on or involving any real estate transaction.

(2) Tangible personal property transactions

My attorney-in-fact may act for me in any manner to deal with all or any part of any interest in personal property that I own at the time of execution of this document or later acquire, under such terms as my attorney-in-fact deems proper. My attorney-in-fact's powers include but are not limited to the power to lease, buy, exchange, accept as a gift or as security for a loan, acquire, possess, maintain, repair, improve, insure, rent, convey, mortgage, pledge, and pay or contest taxes and assessments on any tangible personal property.

(3) Stock and bond, commodity, option and other securities transactions

My attorney-in-fact may do any act which I can do through an agent, with respect to any interest in a bond, share, other instrument of similar character or commodity. My attorney-in-fact's powers include but are not limited to the power to:

(a) Accept as a gift or as security for a loan, reject, demand, buy, receive or otherwise acquire ownership or possession of any bond, share, instrument of similar character, commodity interest or any investment with respect thereto, together with the interest, dividends, proceeds or other distributions connected with it.

(b) Sell (including short sales), exchange, transfer, release, surrender, pledge, trade in or otherwise dispose of any bond, share, instrument of similar character or commodity interest.

(c) Demand, receive and obtain any money or other thing of value to which I am or may become or may claim to be entitled as the proceeds of any interest in a bond, share, other instrument of similar character or commodity interest.

(d) Agree and contract, in any manner, and with any broker or other person and on any terms, for the accomplishment of any purpose listed in this section.

(e) Execute, acknowledge, seal and deliver any instrument my attorney-in-fact thinks useful to accomplish a purpose listed in this section, or any report or certificate required by law or regulation.

(4) *Banking and other financial institution transactions*

My attorney-in-fact may do any act that I can do through an agent in connection with any banking transaction that might affect my financial or other interests. My attorney-in-fact's powers include but are not limited to the power to:

(a) Continue, modify and terminate any deposit account or other banking arrangement, or open either in the name of the agent alone or my name alone or in both our names jointly, a deposit account of any type in any financial institution, rent a safe deposit box or vault space, have access to a safe deposit box or vault to which I would have access, and make other contracts with the institution.

(b) Make, sign and deliver checks or drafts, and withdraw my funds or property from any financial institution by check, order or otherwise.

    (c) Prepare financial statements concerning my assets and liabilities or income and expenses and deliver them to any financial institution, and receive statements, notices or other documents from any financial institution.

    (d) Borrow money from a financial institution on terms my attorney-in-fact deems acceptable, give security out of my assets, and pay, renew or extend the time of payment of any note given by or on my behalf.

(5) Business operating transactions

My attorney-in-fact may do any act that I can do through an agent in connection with any business operated by me that my attorney-in-fact deems desirable. My attorney-in-fact's powers include but are not limited to the power to:

    (a) Perform any duty and exercise any right, privilege or option which I have or claim to have under any contract of partnership, enforce the terms of any partnership agreement, and defend, submit to arbitration or settle any legal proceeding to which I am a party because of membership in a partnership.

    (b) Exercise in person or by proxy and enforce any right, privilege or option which I have as the holder of any bond, share or instrument of similar character and defend, submit to arbitration or settle a legal proceeding to which I am a party because of any such bond, share or instrument of similar character.

    (c) With respect to a business owned solely by me, continue, modify, extend or terminate any contract on my behalf, demand and receive all money that is due or claimed by me and use such funds in the operation of the business, engage in banking transactions my attorney-in-fact deems desirable, determine the location of the operation, the nature of the business it undertakes, its name, methods of manufacturing, selling, marketing, financing, accounting, form of organization and insurance, and hiring and paying employees and independent contractors.

    (d) Execute, acknowledge, seal and deliver any instrument of any kind that my attorney-in-fact thinks useful to accomplish any purpose listed in this section.

(e) Pay, compromise or contest business taxes or assessments.

(f) Demand and receive money or other things of value to which I am or claim to be entitled as the proceeds of any business operation, and conserve, invest, disburse or use anything so received for purposes listed in this section.

(6) *Insurance and annuity transactions*

My attorney-in-fact may do any act that I can do through an agent, in connection with any insurance or annuity policy, that my attorney-in-fact deems desirable. My attorney-in-fact's powers include but are not limited to the power to:

(a) Continue, pay the premium on, modify, rescind or terminate any annuity or policy of life, accident, health, disability or liability insurance procured by me or on my behalf before the execution of this power of attorney. My attorney-in-fact cannot name himself or herself as beneficiary of a renewal, extension or substitute for such a policy unless he or she was already the beneficiary before I signed the power of attorney.

(b) Procure new, different or additional contracts of health, disability, accident or liability insurance on my life, modify, rescind or terminate any such contract and designate the beneficiary of any such contract.

(c) Sell, assign, borrow on, pledge, or surrender and receive the cash surrender value of any policy.

(7) *Estate, trust and other beneficiary transactions*

My attorney-in-fact may act for me in all matters that affect a trust, probate estate, guardianship, conservatorship, escrow, custodianship or other fund from which I am, may become or claim to be entitled, as a beneficiary, to a share or payment. My attorney-in-fact's authority includes the power to disclaim any assets which I am, may become or claim to be entitled, as a beneficiary, to a share or payment.

(8) Living trust transactions

My attorney-in-fact may transfer ownership of any property over which he or she has authority under this document to the trustee of a revocable trust I have created as settlor. Such property may include real property, stocks, bonds, accounts with financial institutions, insurance policies or other property.

(9) Legal actions

My attorney-in-fact may act for me in all matters that affect claims in favor of or against me and proceedings in any court or administrative body. My attorney-in-fact's powers include but are not limited to the power to:

(a) Hire an attorney to assert any claim or defense before any court, administrative board or other tribunal.

(b) Submit to arbitration or mediation or settle any claim in favor of or against me or any litigation to which I am a party, pay any judgment or settlement and receive any money or other things of value paid in settlement.

(10) Personal and family care

My attorney-in-fact may do all acts necessary to maintain my customary standard of living, and that of my spouse and children and other persons customarily supported by or legally entitled to be supported by me. My attorney-in-fact's powers include but are not limited to the power to:

(a) Pay for medical, dental and surgical care, living quarters, usual vacations and travel expenses, shelter, clothing, food, appropriate education and other living costs.

(b) Continue arrangements with respect to automobiles or other means of transportation, charge accounts, discharge of any services or duties assumed by me to any parent, relative or friend, contributions or payments incidental to membership or affiliation in any church, club, society or other organization.

(11) Government benefits

My attorney-in-fact may act for me in all matters that affect my right to government benefits, including Social Security, Medicare, Medicaid, or other governmental programs, or civil or military service. My attorney-in-fact's powers include but are not limited to the power to:

(a) Prepare, execute, file, prosecute, defend, submit to arbitration or settle a claim on my behalf to benefits or assistance, financial or otherwise.

(b) Receive the proceeds of such a claim and conserve, invest, disburse or use them on my behalf.

(12) Retirement plan transactions

My attorney-in-fact may act for me in all matters that affect my retirement plans. My attorney-in-fact's powers include but are not limited to the power to select payment options under any retirement plan in which I participate, make contributions to those plans, exercise investment options, receive payment from a plan, roll over plan benefits into other retirement plans, designate beneficiaries under those plans and change existing beneficiary designations.

(13) Tax matters

My attorney-in-fact may act for me in all matters that affect my local, state and federal taxes. My attorney-in-fact's powers include but are not limited to the power to:

(a) Prepare, sign and file federal, state, local and foreign income, gift, payroll, Federal Insurance Contributions Act returns and other tax returns, claims for refunds, requests for extension of time, petitions, any power of attorney required by the Internal Revenue Service or other taxing authority, and other documents.

(b) Pay taxes due, collect refunds, post bonds, receive confidential information, exercise any election available to me and contest deficiencies determined by a taxing authority.

I understand the importance of the powers I delegate to my attorney-in-fact in this document. I recognize that the document gives my attorney-in-fact broad powers over my assets, and that these powers will become effective as of the date of my incapacity (or sooner if specified in this document) and continue indefinitely unless I revoke this durable power of attorney.

Signed this _____ day of _____, _____
State of Texas, County of _____
Signature: _____
Social Security number: 123-45-6789

WITNESSES

On the date written above, the principal declared to me that this instrument is his durable power of attorney, and that he willingly executed it as a free and voluntary act. The principal signed this instrument in my presence.

Signature: _____

Print Name: _____

Address: _____

Signature: _____

Print Name: _____

Address: _____

CERTIFICATE OF ACKNOWLEDGMENT OF NOTARY PUBLIC

State of Texas   )

) ss.

County of _____)

On _____, _____, before me,

_____, a notary public in and for said

state, personally appeared _____,

personally known to me (or proved on the basis of satisfactory evidence) to be the person whose name is subscribed to the within instrument, and acknowledged to me that he executed the same in his authorized capacity and that by his signature on the instrument the person, or the entity upon behalf of which the person acted, executed the instrument.

                         WITNESS my hand and official seal.

                         _____

                         Notary Public for the

State of Texas

         [NOTARIAL SEAL]   My commission expires: _____

Appendix B: Legal Documents

Delegation of Authority

I, _____, of the

City of _____, County of

_____, State of _____,

am currently serving as attorney-in-fact for

_____ under the durable power of

attorney for finances dated _____.

Under the power granted to me in that document, I delegate the

following authority to _____ for the

period beginning _____ and ending _____

_____

_____

_____

_____

_____

Dated: _____

Signature of Attorney-in-Fact: _____

Name of Attorney-in-Fact: _____

CERTIFICATE OF ACKNOWLEDGMENT OF NOTARY PUBLIC

State of Texas)

) ss.

County of _____)

On _____, _____ before me,

_____, a notary public in and for said state, personally

appeared _____, personally known to me

(or proved on the basis of satisfactory evidence) to be the person whose name is subscribed to the within instrument, and acknowledged to me that she/he executed the same in her/his authorized capacity, and that by her/his signature on the instrument the person, or the entity upon behalf of which the person acted, executed the instrument.

WITNESS my hand and official seal.

_____

Notary Public for the State of Texas

[NOTARIAL SEAL]   My commission expires: _____

Health Care Directive- An Example in the State of Minnesota

INSTRUCTIONS: Health Care Documents

In Minnesota, your written directions for health care are called your Health Care Directive. In addition, Quicken WillMaker produces a notice to your health care providers urging them to carefully read and follow these directions. Your Health Care Directive includes a section in which you may appoint a health care proxy; Minnesota, unlike other states, does not require a separate form such as a durable power of attorney.

Before You Sign

This section lists the steps to take before you finalize your Quicken WillMaker document and put it to use.

Review Your Document

Read your document carefully. Is everything printed as you intended? Do you understand the meaning of every word?

Signing Your Health Care Directive

You must sign and date your Directive in the spaces provided at the end. If you are not able to sign the document, another person may sign for you. You must direct this person to sign and then watch as he or she does so.

Your signature on your Directive must be either witnessed or notarized. Before you sign your document, carefully read and follow the instructions set out below in regard to having your signature witnessed or notarized.

Witnessing Your Health Care Directive

If you choose to have your document witnessed instead of notarized, two people must observe you sign your Directive, but they need not read it. Both witnesses must meet certain qualifications, which are set out in your Directive just above the signature lines. Read these requirements before asking anyone to serve as your witness. Each witness must sign his or her name and print a current address on the lines provided. For an explanation of any unfamiliar terms in the qualifications, see the Quicken WillMaker Legal Manual, Chapter 23.

Notarizing Your Health Care Directive

If you choose to have your Directive notarized rather than witnessed, you must sign it in front of a notary. Take it to the notary and follow his or her instructions. The notary may either sign the notary language on your document or fill in a separate form and attach it to your document. Be prepared to show the notary some identification.

After You Sign

The doctors and other health care personnel attending you must be aware of your written health care directions. The best way to ensure this is to take the IMPORTANT NOTICE—TO MY HEALTH CARE PROVIDER and attach it to your health care directions. Then make several photocopies of your signed, original documents and give one set to each of the following people:

- your regular doctor, if you have one
- the patient representative of your HMO or other medical plan
- the person you name to supervise your health care if you have named one, and
- any other trusted friend or relative.

Place the original with your other valuable papers, such as a will, living trust, deed or insurance policy.

If You Change Your Mind

You may always change your mind and cancel your health care documents. While there are several legal ways to do this, we recommend that you tear up the original documents and all copies. In addition, if your health care provider is aware of your documents, Minnesota law requires that the health care provider be notified of the revocation. As a practical matter, it is always important to inform those who know about your documents that you have revoked it—especially your health care providers and your health care agent, if you have named one. Make sure that all people who have copies of your documents return them to you to be destroyed.

You are not required to revoke your documents in writing, but if you wish to make a written revocation notice to deliver to those who are aware of your health care documents, this program provides a revocation form that you can use.

Understanding Key Terms

The following terms have special meaning when used in your health care directions:

- Terminal condition means an incurable and irreversible condition that will result in death within a relatively short time.
- Permanently unconscious means an unconscious condition from which, to a reasonable degree of medical certainty, there will be no recovery.
- Life-sustaining procedure means any medical procedure, treatment, or intervention which uses mechanical or other artificial means to sustain, restore, or supplant a spontaneous vital function and which would serve to secure only a precarious and burdensome prolongation of life.
- Artificially administered food and water — also called nutrition and hydration — means a mix of nutrients and fluids given through tubes inserted into veins or various body parts, depending on the patient's condition.

Notice to Health Care Provider

IMPORTANT NOTICE
TO MY HEALTH CARE PROVIDER

Please carefully read the attached formal health care document. I have health care instructions that may be different and more extensive than provided for in standardized forms. The attached document contains specific instructions about the health care that I want — or do not want — if I am terminally ill or permanently unconscious and unable to communicate my wishes.

My wishes may be summarized as follows:

If I am terminally ill, I direct that:

- food and water be artificially administered, even if it would also have the effect of prolonging my life.

- medicines and treatments be administered to ease my pain and keep me comfortable.

- all additional life-prolonging procedures be withheld, except the following procedures, which I want provided: blood and blood products, cardio-pulmonary resuscitation (CPR), diagnostic tests and drugs.

If I am permanently unconscious, I direct that:

- food and water be artificially administered, even if it would also have the effect of prolonging my life.

- medicines and treatments be administered to ease my pain and keep me comfortable.

- all additional life-prolonging procedures be withheld, except the following procedures, which I want provided: blood and blood products, cardio-pulmonary resuscitation (CPR), diagnostic tests and drugs.

Thank you for taking the time to understand my health care instructions.
John Doe

Appendix B: Legal Documents

Example HEALTH CARE DIRECTIVE in the State of Minnesota
I, John Doe, understand this document allows me to do one or both of the following.

PART I: Name another person, called the health care agent, to make health care decisions for me if I am unable to decide or speak for myself. My health care agent must make health care decisions for me based on any instructions I provide in Part II.

PART II: Give instructions to guide others making health care decisions for me. If I have named a health care agent, these instructions are to be used by the agent. These instructions may also be used by my health care providers, others assisting with my health care and my family, in the event I cannot make health care decisions for myself.

PART I: APPOINTMENT OF HEALTH CARE AGENT

If I become unable to communicate my instructions, I designate the person named below to act on my behalf consistently with any instructions stated in this document.

My health care agent's power to act expressly includes the authority to:
- hire and fire medical personnel.
- visit me in a hospital or other medical care facility.
- review and receive any information regarding my physical or mental health, including medical and hospital records.
- sign any releases or other documents required to obtain this information.
- sign any documents required to request, withdraw or refuse medical treatment or to be released or transferred from a hospital or other medical facility.
- sign any waiver or release from liability required by a hospital or physician.

I nominate as my health care agent:

Name: Mary Doe

200 At Last Acres
Paradise Valley, Minnesota 55901

Day telephone: 300-572-9132

Evening telephone: 300-672-9173

Relationship: (If any)_____

If the person I have named above refuses or is unable or unavailable to act on my behalf, or if I revoke that person's authority to act as my agent, I authorize the following person to do so:

Name: Bob Doe

    233 Valley Drive
    Paradise Valley, California 03000

Day telephone: 300-256-9243

Evening telephone: 300256-3819

Relationship: (If any)_____

PART II: HEALTH CARE INSTRUCTIONS

Specifically, if I am diagnosed to have a terminal condition, I direct that:

- food and water be artificially administered, even if it would also have the effect of prolonging my life.
- medicines and treatments be administered to ease my pain and keep me comfortable.
- all additional life-prolonging procedures be withheld, except the following procedures, which I want provided: blood and blood products, cardio-pulmonary resuscitation (CPR), diagnostic tests and drugs.

If I am diagnosed to be permanently unconscious, I direct that:

- food and water be artificially administered, even if it would also have the effect of prolonging my life.
- medicines and treatments be administered to ease my pain and keep me comfortable.
- all additional life-prolonging procedures be withheld, except the following procedures, which I want provided: blood and blood products, cardio-pulmonary resuscitation (CPR), diagnostic tests and drugs.

PART III: MAKING THE DOCUMENT LEGAL

SEVERABILITY

If any of the specific directions in this document are held invalid, that shall not affect other directions that can be given effect without the invalid direction.

SIGNATURE

I am thinking clearly, I agree with everything that is written in this document, and I have made this document willingly.

Signed:

_____

Date:

_____

WITNESSES

[Use only if the document is not notarized.]

    Witness #1

Alzheimer's--What My Mother's Caregiving Taught Me

I certify that John Doe, the Declarant, voluntarily signed this Health Care Directive in my presence and that the Declarant is personally known to me. I am not named as agent or alternate agent.

Witness:

_____

Address:

_____

_____

Witness #2

I certify that John Doe, the Declarant, voluntarily signed this Health Care Directive in my presence and that the Declarant is personally known to me. I am not named as agent or alternate agent. And in addition, I am neither a health care provider nor an employee of a health care provider directly attending the Declarant.

Witness:

_____

Address:

_____

_____

NOTARIZATION

[Use only if the document is not witnessed.]

STATE OF _____

COUNTY OF _____

In my presence on _____ (date),

_____ (name) acknowledged his/her signature on this document or acknowledged that he/she authorized the person signing this document to sign on his/her behalf. I am not named as a health care agent or alternate health care agent in this document.

(Signature of Notary) _____   (Notary Stamp)

Notice of Revocation of Health Care Directive

Important: Do not use or sign this document unless you want to revoke your Health Care Directive.

Although Minnesota does not require a written revocation of your Health Care Directive, you can use this document to provide written evidence of your decision to revoke it.

Notice of Revocation of Health Care Directive

I, _____, of the City of
_____, State of
_____, revoke the Health Care Directive dated
_____, empowering
_____ and _____ (as alternate) to make health care decisions for me. I revoke and withdraw all power and authority granted under that document.

Date:

_____

Signature:

_____

Print Name:

_____

Do Not Resuscitate Orders (DNRO)

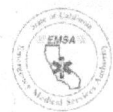

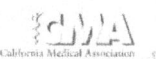

EMERGENCY MEDICAL SERVICES
PREHOSPITAL DO NOT RESUSCITATE (DNR) FORM
An Advance Request to Limit the Scope of Emergency Medical Care

I, _Olive Bublitz_ (print patient's name), request limited emergency care as herein described.

I understand DNR means that if my heart stops beating or if I stop breathing, no medical procedure to restart breathing or heart functioning will be instituted.

I understand this decision will **not** prevent me from obtaining other emergency medical care by prehospital emergency medical care personnel and/or medical care directed by a physician prior to my death.

I understand I may revoke this directive at any time by destroying this form and removing any "DNR" medallions.

I give permission for this information to be given to the prehospital emergency care personnel, doctors, nurses or other health personnel as necessary to implement this directive.

I hereby agree to the "Do Not Resuscitate" (DNR) order.

X _[signature]_   _5/12/06_
Patient/Surrogate Signature   Date

_____
Surrogate's Relationship to Patient

By signing this form, the surrogate acknowledges that this request to forego resuscitative measures is consistent with the known desires of, and with the best interest of, the individual who is the subject of this form.

I affirm that this patient/surrogate is making an informed decision and that this directive is the expressed wish of the patient/surrogate. A copy of this form is in the patient's permanent medical record.

In the event of cardiac or respiratory arrest, no chest compressions, assisted ventilations, intubation, defibrillation, or cardiotonic medications are to be initiated.

[signature]   _5/12/06_
Physician Signature   Date

Razmig Krumian   _818 8899250_
Print Name   Telephone

THIS FORM WILL NOT BE ACCEPTED IF IT HAS BEEN AMENDED OR ALTERED IN ANY WAY

PREHOSPITAL DNR REQUEST FORM

White Copy: To be kept by patient
Yellow Copy: To be kept in patient's permanent medical record
Pink Copy: If authorized DNR medallion desired, submit this form with Medic Alert enrollment form to: Medic Alert Foundation, Turlock, CA 95381

Doctor's Order for Hospice Care

EDWARD B. PORTNOY, M.D.
DEA # AP 6638057   LIC. # G30207(CA)
DARIA M. SCHNEIDMAN, F.N.P., M.N.
DEA # MS 0586113   LIC. # 5701(CA)
PRISCILLA A. LEE, F.N.P., M.N.
DEA # ML 0559231   LIC. # 3592(CA)
1250 LA VENTA ROAD, SUITE 101-B
WESTLAKE VILLAGE, CA 91361-3761
(805) 497-6571 TEL., (805) 497-7082 FAX

NAME _Clive Bushtz_   AGE _8/10/06_

ADDRESS _____   DATE _____

Rx ILLEGAL IF NOT SAFETY BLUE BACKGROUND

℞

Hospice Care
"Alzheimer's Disease"

Buena Vista Hospice

Refill _____ times

DO NOT SUBSTITUTE

To ensure brand name dispensing check and initial box.

♻   5DIM6002232

Final Arrangements-An Example in the State of Florida

Final Arrangements for John Doe

I request that the following instructions and preferences be honored after my death:

Part 1. Body Donation

I have not made arrangements to donate my whole body.

Part 2. Organ Donation

I have not made arrangements for organ donation.

Part 3. Cremation Instructions

A. Mortuary or Crematorium

No preference.

B. Embalming

I do not wish to be embalmed.

C. Casket

No preference.

D. Pre-cremation Ceremony

No ceremony wanted.

E. Witness to Cremation

No preference.

F. Container for Cremated Remains

Brass Urn

G. Burial Site

In Grave with Robert Ernest & Olive May Doe, Roselawn Cemetery, Lake Geneva, Wisconsin

H. Burial Ceremony

No ceremony wanted.

I. Marker

John Doe, Son

J. Epitaph

He Gave His Best To Make World A Better Place and Enjoyed The Best of What Life Has to Offer

K. Memorial Ceremony

No preference.

Part 4. Person to Oversee My Wishes

I want Kathy Doe to oversee the plans I've set out in this document. If Kathy Doe can not serve or be reached when necessary, I want Bob Doe to oversee my plans.

Signature

I, John Doe, declare that I have read these instructions and that they accurately reflect my wishes for final arrangements after my death.

_____   Date: _____

John Doe

Appendix C: Diagnosing Alzheimer's

Alzheimer Association Steps to Diagnosis[70]

- Finding the right doctor
- Understanding the problem
- Reviewing medical history
- Mental status tests
- Physical exam and diagnostic tests
- Neurological exam
- Brain imaging

Finding A House Call Doctor

The first step in following up on symptoms is finding a doctor you feel comfortable with. Alzheimer's Association clients report they are most likely to be satisfied seeing someone who is well informed about Alzheimer's disease. Your local Alzheimer's Association can help you find the right doctor.

There is no single type of doctor who specializes in diagnosing and treating memory loss or Alzheimer's disease. Many people contact their regular primary care physician or internist about their concerns. Primary care doctors often oversee the diagnostic process and provide treatment themselves.

In some cases, the primary care doctor may refer a patient to one of the following specialists:
A neurologist, who specializes in diseases of the brain and nervous system
A psychiatrist, who specializes in disorders that affect mood or the way the mind works
A psychologist with advanced training in testing memory, concentration, problem solving, language and other mental functions

---

[70] Alzheimer's Association National Office 225 N. Michigan Ave., Fl. 17, Chicago, IL 60601 or http://www.alz.org.

Understanding the problem

There is no single test that proves a person has Alzheimer's. The medical workup is designed to evaluate overall health and identify any conditions that could affect how well the mind works.

Experts estimate a skilled physician can diagnose Alzheimer's with more than 90 percent accuracy. Doctors can almost always determine that a person has dementia, but it may sometimes be difficult to pin down the exact cause.

Be prepared for the doctor to ask:
- What kind of symptoms have you noticed?
- When did they begin?
- How often do they happen?
- Have they gotten worse?

Dementia screening tests

An increasing number of test developers, health care facilities and others are marketing dementia screening tests directly to consumers. The Alzheimer's Association believes that home screening tests can not and should not be used as a substitute for a thorough examination by a skilled doctor. There is an established diagnostic criteria that physicians adhere to when evaluating someone for Alzheimer's disease.

Although dementia screening tests don't claim to offer a definitive diagnosis, any test that plants the idea of a serious illness has the potential to cause great psychological distress to the test taker. The whole process of assessment and diagnosis should be carried out within the context of an ongoing relationship with responsible health care professionals.

Reviewing medical history

The doctor will interview the person being examined or family members to gather information about current and past illnesses. The doctor will also obtain a history of medical conditions affecting other family members, especially whether they may have had Alzheimer's disease or a related disorder.

It is helpful to bring a list of all the medications the person is taking. The doctor will obtain a history of key medical conditions affecting other family members, especially whether they may have had Alzheimer's disease or related disorders.

Mental status tests

Mental status testing gives the doctor a general idea of whether a person:

- Is aware of having symptoms or feels nothing is wrong

- Knows the date, time and where he or she is

- Can remember a short list of words, follow instructions and do simple calculations

Mini-mental state exam (MMSE)

The mini-mental state examination (MMSE) is one of the tests most commonly used to assess mental function. In the MMSE, a health professional asks a patient a series of questions designed to test a range of everyday mental skills.

Examples of questions include:

- Remember and repeat a few minutes later the names of three common objects (for instance, horse, flower, penny)

- State the year, season, day of the week and date

- Count backward from 100 by 7s or spell "world" backwards

- Name two familiar objects present in the office as the examiner points to them

- Identify the location of the examiner's office (state, city, street address, floor)

- Repeat a common phrase or saying after the examiner

- Copy a picture of two interlocking shapes

- Follow a three-part instruction, such as: take a piece of paper in your right hand, fold it in half, and place it on the floor

The maximum MMSE score is 30 points. A score of 20 - 24 suggests mild dementia, 13 - 20 suggests moderate dementia, and less than 12 indicates severe dementia. On average, the MMSE score of a person with Alzheimer's declines about 2 - 4 points each year.

Mini-cog

Another popular mental status test is the "mini-cog," which involves two tasks: (1) remembering and a few minutes later repeating the names of three common objects, and (2) drawing a face of a clock showing all 12 numbers in the right places and a time specified by the examiner.

In addition to assessing mental status, the doctor will evaluate a person's sense of well-being to detect depression or other mood disorders that can cause memory problems, loss of interest in life, and other symptoms that can overlap with dementia.

Physical Exam and Diagnostic Tests

The physician will:

- Ask about diet, nutrition and use of alcohol.
- Review all medications. It is helpful to bring a list or the containers of all medicines currently being taken, including over-the-counter drugs and supplements.
- Check blood pressure, temperature and pulse.
- Listen to the heart and lungs.
- Collect samples of blood and urine.

Information from these tests can help identify other disorders that may cause memory loss, confused thinking, trouble focusing attention, or other symptoms similar to dementia. Such disorders include:

- Anemia, malnutrition or certain vitamin deficiencies
- Excess use of alcohol
- Medication side effects
- Certain infections
- Diabetes
- Kidney or liver disease
- Thyroid abnormalities
- Problems with the heart, lung or blood vessels

Neurological exam

The neurological examination is an important part of the physical. Its goal is to assess the function of the brain and nervous system to identify symptoms of brain disorders other than Alzheimer's.

During the neurological exam, the physician may test:

- Reflexes
- Coordination and balance
- Muscle tone and strength
- Eye movement
- Speech
- Sensation

Brain Imaging

New imaging technologies have revolutionized our understanding of the structure and function of the living brain.

Structural imaging provides information about the shape, position or volume of brain tissue. Structural techniques include magnetic resonance imaging (MRI) and computed tomography (CT).
Functional imaging reveals how well cells in various brain regions are working by showing how actively the cells use sugar or oxygen. Functional techniques include positron emission tomography (PET) and functional MRI (MRI).

Currently, a standard medical workup for Alzheimer's disease often includes structural imaging with MRI or, less frequently, CT. These images are used primarily to detect tumors, evidence of small or large strokes, damage from severe head trauma or a buildup of fluid.

Promising areas for brain imaging research

Researchers are studying whether the use of MRI and other imaging methods may be expanded to play a more direct role in diagnosing Alzheimer's. Many studies have shown that the brains of people with Alzheimer's shrink significantly as the disease progresses.

Research has also shown that shrinkage in specific brain regions may be an early sign of Alzheimer's. However, scientists have not yet agreed upon standardized values that would establish the significance of a specific amount of shrinkage for any individual person at a single point in time.

Research with PET and other functional imaging methods also suggests that those with Alzheimer's typically have reduced brain cell activity in certain regions. However, as with the shrinkage detected by structural imaging, there is not yet enough information to translate these general patterns of reduced activity into diagnostic information about individuals.

At this time, PET is used primarily in research studies in hopes of gaining further knowledge about its potential for wider use in diagnosing Alzheimer's and monitoring progression and response to treatment.

Today, Medicare will cover a PET scan for Alzheimer's only to help distinguish the disease from frontotemporal dementia, a rare related disorder that may cause dramatic loss of function in the front and side regions of the brain.

Another promising area of functional imaging research focuses on developing tracer compounds that will attach to key abnormal brain deposits implicated in Alzheimer's. For example, preliminary data suggests that one such tracer, called Pittsburgh compound B, may attach to beta-amyloid and "light up" in a PET scan.

Mayo Clinic Specialist Interview on Alzheimer's

To diagnose Alzheimer's disease, doctors rule out several other conditions and recommend psychological testing. "It's tough but worth the effort," says a Mayo Clinic specialist.[71]

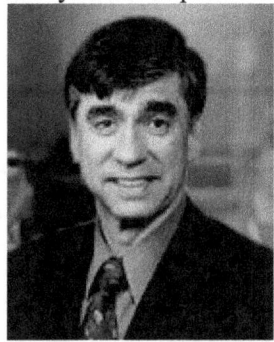

Eric Tangalos, M.D.

In this interview, Eric Tangalos, M.D., a primary care physician and geriatrician affiliated with the Alzheimer's Disease Research Center at Mayo Clinic, Rochester, Minn., explains why older people with memory problems should have a thorough diagnostic workup. If fears are confirmed, information and planning can smooth the path for the ensuing years.

Is an autopsy of the brain the only way to diagnose Alzheimer's disease?

Many people believe that you have to have the brain at autopsy before you can diagnose Alzheimer's, but that's not right. We do that for research, to confirm the diagnosis, but we can also identify the disease clinically with time and other tests.

A two- to four-hour battery of neuropsychological tests is a routine part of our Alzheimer's research at Mayo Clinic. We compare skill levels of people who may have Alzheimer's with those of people at the same age and

---

[71] Eric Tangalos, M.D., primary care physician and co-director for education at the Alzheimer's Disease Research Center, The Mayo Clinic, Rochester, MN, December 5. 2006, http://www.mayoclinic.com/health/alzheimers/AZ00017.

education level. We know that an 85-year-old is not going to function as well as a 75-year-old. These tests show us exactly what people can and cannot do based on comparisons to standard tests of people with the same sex, education and age.

Could you describe these neuropsychological tests?

These are mental tests that look at different functions in the brain. Different parts of the brain do different things. Language can be affected, or problem solving. These tests break down the functions of the brain into more basic elements. Short-term memory is different from long-term memory. Performing calculations is different from remembering words. Drawing pictures is different from working through a maze.

Figuring out what a person can and cannot do not only helps establish the right diagnosis, but also helps determine what the individual is still capable of doing either at work or at home. From these studies and knowing what support they have at home, we can tell if the person can still function independently or if he or she is really on the edge and should be looking for a safer living environment.

Does everyone have to go through a battery of tests?

It is a good idea to have a full evaluation when contemplating the diagnosis. I tell people that there's not a better investment in time or effort. There are lots of brief tests that can be done in the office, but they can only screen for disease and may miss a problem altogether. Longer cognitive tests are more thorough and provide information that has greater accuracy.

How can people recognize the early signs of Alzheimer's?

In the earliest stage of the disease, a diagnosis can be really difficult. What you're looking for is something that doesn't fit with the individual's former level of function. That's why family members often notice the symptoms first. The disease is more than just memory — it can involve language, problem solving or even how we draw a clock.

It's easy to misplace your car in the parking lot. That's happened to all of us. But most of us eventually find our cars. People with Alzheimer's lose the capacity to adjust and solve the problem of the lost car. In fact, they might jump to the conclusion that the car has been stolen.

Alzheimer's is a progressive disease that first manifests itself with problems usually related to memory. Over time, people have more difficulty with tasks. By the end of the disease process, Alzheimer's is pretty easy to recognize. Our goal is to find out from family as quickly as possible when something is truly amiss in order to do something about it.

What are the warning signs of Alzheimer's disease?
The Alzheimer's Association's 10 warning signs are:
1. Memory loss
2. Difficulty performing familiar tasks
3. Problems with language
4. Disorientation to time and place
5. Poor or decreased judgment
6. Problems with abstract thinking
7. Misplacing things
8. Changes in mood or behavior
9. Changes in personality
10. Loss of initiative

At what point in the disease are most people getting diagnosed?
There are three broad stages of Alzheimer's. The first stage is cognitive decline, the second stage is functional decline and the third stage is behavioral decline — which usually occurs during the last three years of the person's life.

Most people come in during the second stage, when they are having trouble balancing a checkbook or are getting lost. It's gotten to the point that something has to be done.

Why don't people go to their doctor sooner?
There remains a tremendous anxiety regarding Alzheimer's. They want to blame aging even when they can tell that other people their age aren't having the same difficulties. People hide their symptoms, or spouses cover for them. There's a fear of losing control. They don't want to give up their driving privileges or go in a nursing home. But just because you have a memory problem doesn't mean you can't drive a car. We look for what you have retained as well as what you may have lost.

Do some doctors hesitate to make an Alzheimer's diagnosis?
Many doctors still believe that an early diagnosis of Alzheimer's would overwhelm both families and physicians. It takes a lot of time and effort to manage the disease, both from the person's family and from his or her physician. That's why the Alzheimer's Association tries to provide resources in the community.

I like to use the Alzheimer's word sooner rather than later. I don't want my patients or families to hide from it. We believe in diagnostic disclosure because we think there is a lot that can be done for the problem and that the sooner it is recognized, the more we have available as treatment options.

Today, I think we're talking about Alzheimer's as openly as we were starting to talk about cancer 30 years ago and about depression 10 to 15 years ago. It's a real disease, long before it prevents a person from functioning, and we need to do something about it.

Can magnetic resonance imaging (MRI) or computerized tomography (CT) scans help in diagnosing Alzheimer's?

There's no biological marker that shows someone has the disease. The brain typically changes with Alzheimer's, and those changes can be pretty specific and show up on imaging tests. But that's not enough to make a diagnosis. There's a lot of overlap in what we consider normal and abnormal, so even if some areas change on CT or MRI, the person may still function quite well.

In our research, we use brain changes on MRI to help us confirm the possibility of Alzheimer's. In most clinical settings, brain imaging should be used only to rule out such things as hemorrhages, brain tumors or strokes.

What other diseases should be ruled out?

We'd want to check the thyroid, to rule out problems there. And, in many cases, the symptoms of depression can be mistaken for Alzheimer's — and vice versa. We also routinely look for vitamin B-12 deficiency and always try to make sure that the person is generally healthy and doesn't have some other serious medical problem that would complicate our diagnosis. A lot of our older patients have other medical problems that just make things worse — like heart disease, diabetes, kidney disease, lung disease or any combination of these.

Do people need to be referred to a neurologist?

Most of the doctors treating Alzheimer's are primary care physicians. I've asked neurologists for help with a diagnosis, especially with younger patients. But many people, particularly frail older adults, can't get to any medical center with specialists. It's just too hard for them to travel.

The problems facing people with Alzheimer's are issues of society and economy, and these are best handled by a primary care physician, as long as there are resources in the community to help and the doctor has a true interest in understanding the disease and his or her patients with it.

What's the benefit of an early diagnosis?

There are both drug and nondrug interventions, and everything works best in the earliest stages of disease.

How much do Alzheimer's drugs help?

Drug therapy is only modestly effective. It's not a magic bullet, but it can delay or slow the progress of the disease. It's not like taking an antibiotic and seeing your fever go away, or taking a diuretic and losing 10 pounds. Alzheimer's drugs help some people more than others, but in general, you end up better on the drugs than not on them. With this disease right now, "better" is just not getting worse.

If drugs don't help much, why get diagnosed early?

An early diagnosis isn't just about starting drug therapy. You can change your home environment and simplify the world around you. A lot can be done to make the environment easier for a person with Alzheimer's. I'm a big fan of motion detectors. They're inexpensive and can be very handy in the bathroom or on the back staircase. They do the thinking for you, and when attached to a light switch, they turn on a light even before it comes to mind to do it yourself.

You might choose to have a phone with big push buttons. You can put photos of whom you're calling on the appropriate speed-dial buttons. You can also make small adjustments to improve communication. For example, it's difficult for people with Alzheimer's to concentrate on what is being said if there's noise, like a TV, in the background. The solution is simple: Turn off the TV before you talk.

What else can be done?

People with Alzheimer's do better when they have a routine. It allows them to refresh and reinforce their pattern of behavior every day. They get to relearn their habits over and over and this is good.

When you put them in strange surroundings, they don't do well. That's why they may have trouble when you bring them to your house for the holidays, or if they have to be hospitalized. A change in routine is not good for people with Alzheimer's — there are just too many problems to try and solve.

Alzheimer's--What My Mother's Caregiving Taught Me

The change in routine is one of the reasons why people with Alzheimer's often have such a swift downturn after the death of a spouse. The spouse may have been helping to both think for and protect the person.

Are there other benefits of early diagnosis?

The earlier you're diagnosed, the more capable you are of deciding how you want the rest of your life to be structured. Predictable routines will help you succeed instead of fail.

The sooner you move into a structured environment, the more protected you'll be. The ideal setting is probably one that includes independent housing, assisted living and nursing services on the same campus. The same philosophy is at play throughout, so there's less to learn with each move.

I tell people to move early or late, but not in the middle stages of their disease. Each move will result in a decline in the person's retained abilities. In the early stages, the person can adjust to it better. And in the late stages, their function is already extremely impaired. The middle stage is where we can still try to keep the patient from really losing ground, and a move at this time causes the disease to deteriorate even further.

The problem is that most people don't get diagnosed with Alzheimer's until they reach the middle stage. If you move them during this middle stage, their function declines and it doesn't come back.

Is there anything people can do to reduce their risk?

There's a close link between Alzheimer's and vascular disease. Baby boomers who are concerned about maintaining their brains should take care of their blood vessels as well. That means exercise, which helps keep your blood pressure and weight down. There's also emerging evidence that exercising your brain with socialization and tasks might help.

What do you hope to see in the future?

I'd like to see people come in earlier for diagnosis. The real problem is that they're coming too late. That's easy to understand because Alzheimer's is such a devastating disease. But we'd like patients and families to run toward a diagnosis, rather than away from it.

Laboratory Evaluation of Dementia[72]

TEST	INTENDED DIAGNOSIS	USE	COMMENTS
Psychometric testing	All dementias, especially MCI, FTD	In appropriate clinical context	Virtually required for MCI, mild AD, and FTD; may be essential if medicolegal complications are possible
CBC, electrolyte panel, calcium, SUN, creatinine, glucose	Common metabolic disorders	Routinely	Not intended to be dementia-specific, but part of routine screening for any elderly person
Vitamin B12	Vitamin B12 deficiency	Routinely	Common disorder in elderly persons; may be associated with cognitive impairment
Thyrotropin	Hypothyroidism	Routinely	Common disorder in elderly persons; may be associated with cognitive impairment
MRI or CT (most clinicians prefer MRI when imaging is	Brain structural lesions; CJD	Routinely, in certain circumstances	Needed only at initial diagnosis or after a rapid clinical change; perfusion MRI for CJD

[72] Ronald C. Petersen, M.D., Ph.D.; David S. Knopman, M.D.; and Bradley F. Boeve, M.D., "Essentials of the Proper Diagnosis of Mild Cognitive Impairment, Dementia, and Major Subtypes of Dementia." Mayo Clinic Proceedings 2003; 78: 1290-1308.

TEST	INTENDED DIAGNOSIS	USE	COMMENTS
indicated)			
PET or SPECT	AD, FTD	For added diagnostic certainty in selected cases	Marginal additive value over clinical diagnosis for AD; perhaps more helpful in FTD
EEG	CJD	When CJD is suspected	Not useful routinely, but required as part of a diagnosis for CJD
APOE genotyping	AD	Rarely	Marginal additive value over clinical diagnosis; not recommended for risk prediction
Standard CSF analysis	Meningitis, meningeal cancer, encephalitis	In rapidly progressive dementias	None
CSF analysis for 14-3-3 protein or neuronspecific enolase	CJD	When CJD is suspected	Highly sensitive and specific, if acute infections, stroke, and neoplastic diseases are excluded by other means
CSF analysis for betaamyloid and tau	AD	Rarely	Marginal additive value over clinical diagnosis

Note: AD = Alzheimer's disease; APOE = apolipoprotein E; CBC = complete blood count; CJD = Creutzfeldt-Jakob disease; CSF = cerebrospinal fluid; CT = computed tomography; EEG = electroencephalography; FTD = frontotemporal dementia; MCI = mild cognitive impairment; MRI = magnetic resonance imaging; PET = positron emission tomography; SPECT = single-photon emission CT; SUN = serum urea nitrogen.

Understanding Stages & Symptoms of Alzheimer

Alzheimer Association Description of Stages and Symptoms of Alzheimer's

Stage 1: No impairment

Normal function.

- Unimpaired individuals experience no memory problems and none are evident to a health care professional during a medical interview.

Stage 2: Very mild cognitive decline

May be normal age-related or earliest Alzheimer's sign. Individuals may feel as if they have memory lapses, especially in forgetting familiar words or names or the location of keys, eyeglasses or other everyday objects. But these problems are not evident during a medical examination or apparent to friends, family or co-workers.

Stage 3: Mild cognitive decline

Early-stage Alzheimer's can be diagnosed in some, but not all, individuals with these symptoms. Friends, family or co-workers begin to notice deficiencies. Problems with memory or concentration may be measurable in clinical testing or discernible during a detailed medical interview. Common difficulties include:

- Word- or name-finding problems noticeable to family or close associates
- Decreased ability to remember names when introduced to new people
- Performance issues in social or work settings noticeable to family, friends or co-workers
- Reading a passage and retaining little material
- Losing or misplacing a valuable object
- Decline in ability to plan or organize

Stage 4: Moderate cognitive decline

Mild or early-stage Alzheimer's disease. At this stage, a careful medical interview detects clear-cut deficiencies in the following areas:
Decreased knowledge of recent occasions or current events

- Impaired ability to perform challenging mental arithmetic-for example, to count backward from 75 by 7s
- Decreased capacity to perform complex tasks, such as planning dinner for guests, paying bills and managing finances
- Reduced memory of personal history
- The affected individual may seem subdued and withdrawn, especially in socially or mentally challenging situations

Stage 5: Moderately severe cognitive decline

Moderate or mid-stage Alzheimer's disease. Major gaps in memory and deficits in cognitive function emerge. Some assistance with day-to-day activities becomes essential. At this stage, individuals may:

- Be unable during a medical interview to recall such important details as their current address, their telephone number or the name of the college or high school from which they graduated
- Become confused about where they are or about the date, day of the week or season
- Have trouble with less challenging mental arithmetic; for example, counting backward from 40 by 4s or from 20 by 2s
- Need help choosing proper clothing for the season or the occasion
- Usually retain substantial knowledge about themselves and know their own name and the names of their spouse or children
- Usually require no assistance with eating or using the toilet

Stage 6: Severe cognitive decline

Moderately severe or mid-stage Alzheimer's disease. Memory difficulties continue to worsen, significant personality changes may emerge and affected individuals need extensive help with customary daily activities. At this stage, individuals may:

- Lose most awareness of recent experiences and events as well as of their surroundings
- Recollect their personal history imperfectly, although they generally recall their own name

- Occasionally forget the name of their spouse or primary caregiver but generally can distinguish familiar from unfamiliar faces
- Need help getting dressed properly; without supervision, may make such errors as putting pajamas over daytime clothes or shoes on wrong feet
- Experience disruption of their normal sleep/waking cycle
- Need help with handling details of toileting (flushing toilet, wiping and disposing of tissue properly)
- Have increasing episodes of urinary or fecal incontinence
- Experience significant personality changes and behavioral symptoms, including suspiciousness and delusions (for example, believing that their caregiver is an impostor); hallucinations (seeing or hearing things that are not really there); or compulsive, repetitive behaviors such as hand-wringing or tissue shredding
- Tend to wander and become lost

Stage 7: Very severe cognitive decline

Severe or late-stage Alzheimer's disease. This is the final stage of the disease when individuals lose the ability to respond to their environment, the ability to speak and, ultimately, the ability to control movement.

- Frequently individuals lose their capacity for recognizable speech, although words or phrases may occasionally be uttered
- Individuals need help with eating and toileting and there is general incontinence of urine
- Individuals lose the ability to walk without assistance, then the ability to sit without support, the ability to smile, and the ability to hold their head up. Reflexes become abnormal and muscles grow rigid. Swallowing is impaired.

Later Stage Changes [73]
Mild AD (Similar to Stage 4 above)

- Loses spark or zest for life - does not start anything.
- Loses recent memory without a change in appearance or casual conversation.
- Loses judgment about money.
- Has difficulty with new learning and making new memories.
- Has trouble finding words - may substitute or make up words that sound like or mean something like the forgotten word.
- May stop talking to avoid making mistakes.
- Has shorter attention span and less motivation to stay with an activity.
- Easily loses way going to familiar places.
- Resists change or new things.
- Has trouble organizing and thinking logically.
- Asks repetitive questions.
- Withdraws, loses interest, is irritable, not as sensitive to others' feelings, uncharacteristically angry when frustrated or tired.
- Won't make decisions. For example, when asked what she wants to eat, says "I'll have what she is having."
- Takes longer to do routine chores and becomes upset if rushed or if something unexpected happens.
- Forgets to pay, pays too much, or forgets how to pay - may hand the checkout person a wallet instead of the correct amount of money.
- Forgets to eat, eats only one kind of food, or eats constantly.
- Loses or misplaces things by hiding them in odd places or forgets where things go, such as putting clothes in the dishwasher.

---

[73] Adapted from Caring for People with Alzheimer's Disease: A Manual for Facility Staff, 2nd edition, by Lisa P. Gwyther, 2001. Published by the American Health Care Association, 1201 L Street, NW, Washington, DC 20005 and the Alzheimer's Association, 919 N. Michigan Ave., Suite 1100, Chicago, IL 60611.

- Constantly checks, searches or hoards things of no value.

Moderate AD (Similar to Stage 5 above)

- Changes in behavior, concern for appearance, hygiene, and sleep become more noticeable.
- Mixes up identity of people, such as thinking a son is a brother or that a wife is a stranger.
- Poor judgment creates safety issues when left alone - may wander and risk exposure, poisoning, falls, self-neglect or exploitation.
- Has trouble recognizing familiar people and own objects; may take things that belong to others.
- Continuously repeats stories, favorite words, statements, or motions like tearing tissues.
- Has restless, repetitive movements in late afternoon or evening, such as pacing, trying doorknobs, fingering draperies.
- Cannot organize thoughts or follow logical explanations.
- Has trouble following written notes or completing tasks.
- Makes up stories to fill in gaps in memory. For example might say, "Mama will come for me when she gets off work."
- May be able to read but cannot formulate the correct response to a written request.
- May accuse, threaten, curse, fidget or behave inappropriately, such as kicking, hitting, biting, screaming or grabbing.
- May become sloppy or forget manners.
- May see, hear, smell, or taste things that are not there.
- May accuse spouse of an affair or family members of stealing.
- Naps frequently or awakens at night believing it is time to go to work.
- Has more difficulty positioning the body to use the toilet or sit in a chair.
- May think mirror image is following him or television story is happening to her.

- Needs help finding the toilet, using the shower, remembering to drink, and dressing for the weather or occasion.
- Exhibits inappropriate sexual behavior, such as mistaking another individual for a spouse.
- Forgets what is private behavior
- May disrobe or masturbate in public.

Common Changes in Severe AD (Similar to Stage 6 & 7 above)

- Doesn't recognize self or close family.
- Speaks in gibberish, is mute, or is difficult to understand.
- May refuse to eat, chokes, or forgets to swallow.
- May repetitively cry out, pat or touch everything.
- Loses control of bowel and bladder.
- Loses weight and skin becomes thin and tears easily.
- May look uncomfortable or cry out when transferred or touched.
- Forgets how to walk or is too unsteady or weak to stand alone.
- May have seizures, frequent infections, falls.
- May groan, scream or mumble loudly.
- Sleeps more.
- Needs total assistance for all activities of daily living.

Appendix D: Alzheimer Disease Research Centers

Arizona

Arizona Alzheimer's Disease Center/Sun Health Research Institute
Eric Reiman, M.D., Director
Arizona Alzheimer's Disease Center
Banner Alzheimer's Institute
901 E. Willeta Street
Phoenix, AZ 85006
Website: www.azalz.org/
Information Line: 602-239-6525
Director's e-mail: eric.reiman@bannerhealth.com
Director's Tel: 602-239-6999
Director's Fax: 602-239-6253

California

University of California, Davis
Charles S. DeCarli, M.D., Director
Alzheimer's Disease Center
University of California, Davis Medical Center
4860 Y Street, Suite 3700
Sacramento, CA 95817-4540
Website: http://alzheimer.ucdavis.edu
Information Line: 916-734-5496
Director's e-mail: cdecarli@ucdavis.edu
Fax: 916-734-6525

University of California, Irvine
Carl W. Cotman, Ph.D., Director
Alzheimer's Disease Research Center
University of California, Irvine
Gillespie Neuroscience Research Facility, Rm. 1113
Irvine, CA 92697-4540
Website: www.alz.uci.edu
Information Line: 949-824-5847
Director's e-mail: cwcotman@uci.edu
Director's Tel: 949-824-5847

Director's Fax: 949-824-2071

University of California, Los Angeles
Jeffrey L. Cummings, M.D., Director
Alzheimer's Disease Center
10911 Weyburn Avenue, Ste. 200
Los Angeles, CA 90095-1769
Website: www.adc.ucla.edu
Information Line: 310-794-3665
Director's e-mail: jcummings@mednet.ucla.edu
Director's Tel: 310-794-3665
Director's Fax: 310-794-3148

University of California, San Diego
Douglas R. Galasko, M.D., Director
Alzheimer's Disease Research Center
Department of Neurosciences
UCSD School of Medicine
9500 Gilman Drive (0948)
La Jolla, CA 92093-0948
Website: http://adrc.ucsd.edu
Information Line: 858-622-5800
ADC e-mail: adrc@ucsd.edu
Director's e-mail: dgalasko@ucsd.edu
Center Fax: 858-622-1017

University of California, San Francisco
Bruce Miller, M.D., Director
Alzheimer's Disease Research Center
University of California, San Francisco, Box 1207
350 Parnassus Avenue, Suite 905
San Francisco, CA 94143-1207
Website: http://memory.ucsf.edu
Information Line: 415-476-6880
ADC e-mail: adrc@memory.ucsf.edu
Director's e-mail: bmiller@memory.ucsf.edu
Director's Tel: 415-476-5569
Director's Fax: 415-476-4800

Appendix D: Alzheimer's Disease Research Centers Directory

University of Southern California
Helena Chui, M.D., Director
Alzheimer's Disease Research Center
University of Southern California
Health Consultation Center
1510 San Pablo Street, HCC643
Los Angeles, CA 90033
Website: www.usc.edu/dept/gero/ADRC
Information Line: 323-442-7600
ADC e-mail: uscadrc@usc.edu
Director's e-mail: chui@usc.edu
Director's Tel: 323-442-7686
Director's Fax: 323-442-7689

Florida

Florida Alzheimer's Disease Research Center/Byrd Alzheimer's Institute
Huntington Potter, Ph.D., Director
Florida Alzheimer's Disease Research Center
Byrd Alzheimer's Institute
4001 East Fletcher Avenue
Tampa, FL 33613
Website: www.floridaadrc.org
Information Line: 1-866-700-7773 (toll free)
Director's email: hpotter@byrdinstitute.org
Director's Tel: 813-866-1600
Director's Fax: 813-866-1601

Georgia

Emory University
Allan I. Levey, M.D., Ph.D., Director
Alzheimer's Disease Center
Wesley Woods Health Center, 3rd Floor
1841 Clifton Road
Atlanta, GA 30329
Website: www.med.emory.edu/ADC
Information Line: 404-728-6950
Director's e-mail: alevey@emory.edu
Director's Tel: 404-727-7220
Fax: 404-727-3999

Illinois

Northwestern University
M. Marsel Mesulam, M.D., Director
Cognitive Neurology and Alzheimer's Disease Center
Feinberg School of Medicine
Northwestern University
675 N St. Claire, Galter 20-100
Chicago, IL 60611
Website: www.brain.northwestern.edu
Information Line: 312-908-9339
Director's e-mail: mmesulam@northwestern.edu
Director's Tel: 312-908-9339
Director's Fax: 312-908-8789

Rush University Medical Center
David A. Bennett, M.D., Director
Alzheimer's Disease Center
Rush University Medical Center
Armour Academic Center
600 South Paulina Street, Suite 1028
Chicago, IL 60612
Website: www.rush.edu/radc
Information Line: 312-942-3333
Director's e-mail: dbennett@rush.edu
Center's Fax: 312-563-4605

Indiana

Indiana University
Bernardino Ghetti, M.D., Director
Indiana Alzheimer Disease Center
Department of Pathology and Lab Medicine
Indiana University School of Medicine
635 Barnhill Drive, MS-A-138
Indianapolis, IN 46202-5120
Website: http://iadc.iupui.edu
Information Line: 317-278-5500
ADC e-mail: iadc@iupui.edu
Director's e-mail: bghetti@iupui.edu
Director's Tel: 317-274-7818

Director's Fax: 317-274-4882

Kentucky

University of Kentucky
William R. Markesbery, M.D., Director
University of Kentucky Alzheimer's Disease Center
Sanders-Brown Center on Aging, Rm. 101
800 South Limestone St.
Lexington, KY 40536-0230
Website: www.mc.uky.edu/coa/
Information Line: 859-323-6040
Director's e-mail: wmark0@email.uky.edu
Fax: 859-323-2866

Maryland

The Johns Hopkins University
Donald L. Price, M.D., Director
Alzheimer's Disease Research Center
Division of Neuropathology
The Johns Hopkins University Medical Institutions
558 Ross Research Building
720 Rutland Avenue
Baltimore, MD 21205-2196
Website: www.alzresearch.org
Information Line: 410-502-5164
Director's e-mail: priced@jhmi.edu
Director's Tel: 410-502-5169
Director's Fax: 410-955-9777

Massachusetts

Boston University
Neil William Kowall, M.D., Director
Alzheimer's Disease Center
Bedford VA Medical Center
GRECC Program (182B)
200 Springs Road
Bedford, MA 01730
Website: www.bu.edu/alzresearch
Information Line: 1-888-458-2823 (toll free)
ADC e-mail: decart@bu.edu

Director's e-mail: nkowall@bu.edu
Director's Tel: 781-687-2632
Director's Fax: 781-687-3515

Massachusetts General Hospital/Harvard Medical School
Bradley T. Hyman, M.D., Ph.D., Director
Alzheimer's Disease Research Center
Massachusetts General Hospital
114 16th Street, Room 2009
Charlestown, MA 02129
Website: http://madrc.org
Information Line: 617-726-3987
Director's e-mail: b_hyman@helix.mgh.harvard.edu
Director's Tel: 617-726-2299
Director's Fax: 617-724-1480

Michigan

University of Michigan
Sid Gilman, M.D., Director
Alzheimer's Disease Research Center
Department of Neurology
300 North Ingalls, Room 3D15
Ann Arbor, MI 48109-0489
Website: www.med.umich.edu/alzheimers
Information Line: 734-764-2190
ADC e-mail: neuro-ADresearch@med.umich.edu
Director's e-mail: sgilman@umich.edu
Director's Tel: 734-936-1808
Director's Fax: 734-763-1752

Minnesota

Mayo Clinic
Ronald Petersen, M.D., Ph.D., Director
Alzheimer's Disease Research Center
4111 Highway 52 North
Rochester, MN 55901
Website: http://mayoresearch.mayo.edu/mayo/research/alzheimers_center
Information Line: 507-284-1324
ADC e-mail: mayoADC@mayo.edu
Director's e-mail: peter8@mayo.edu

Director's Tel: 507-538-0487
Director's Fax: 507-284-6012
Main Fax: 507-538-0878

Missouri

Washington University
John C. Morris, M.D., Director
Alzheimer's Disease Research Center
Washington University School of Medicine
Department of Neurology
4488 Forest Park Avenue, Suite 130
St. Louis, MO 63108-2293
Website: http://alzheimer.wustl.edu
Information Line: 314-286-2881
Director's e-mail: morrisj@abraxas.wustl.edu
Director's Tel: 314-286-2881
Director's Fax: 314-286-2763

New York

Columbia University
Michael L. Shelanski, M.D., Ph.D., Director
Columbia University Alzheimer's Disease Center
630 West 168th Street, P&S 15-402
New York, NY 10032
Website: www.alzheimercenter.org
Information Line: 212-305-1818
Director's e-mail: mls7@columbia.edu
Director's Tel: 212-305-3300
Director's Fax: 212-305-5498

Mount Sinai School of Medicine
Mary Sano, Ph.D., Director
Alzheimer's Disease Research Center
Department of Psychiatry
Mount Sinai School of Medicine
One Gustave Levy Place, Box 1230
New York, NY 10029-6574
Website: www.mssm.edu/psychiatry/adrc
Information Line: 212-241-8329
Director's e-mail: mary.sano@mssm.edu

Director's Tel: 718-741-4228
Fax: 718-562-9120

New York University
Steven H. Ferris, Ph.D., Director
Alzheimer's Disease Center
New York University
ADRC, Millhauser Labs
560 First Avenue
New York, NY 10016
Website: www.med.nyu.edu/adc
Information Line: 212-263-8088
Director's e-mail: steven.ferris@med.nyu.edu
Director's Tel: 212-263-5703
Director's Fax: 212-263-6991

North Carolina

Duke University Medical Center
Kathleen A. Welsh-Bohmer, Ph.D., Director
Joseph and Kathleen Bryan Alzheimer's Disease Research Center
2200 West Main Street
Suite A-200
Durham, NC 27705
Website: http://adrc.mc.duke.edu
Information Line: 1-866-444-2372 (toll free)
Director's e-mail: kwe@duke.edu
Director's Tel: 919-668-1553
Director's Fax: 919-668-0828

Oregon

Oregon Health and Science University
Jeffrey Kaye, M.D., Director
Aging and Alzheimer's Disease Center CR 131
Oregon Health and Science University
3181 SW Sam Jackson Park Road
Portland, OR 97239-3098
Website: www.ohsu.edu/research/alzheimers
Information Line: 503-494-6976
Director's e-mail: kaye@ohsu.edu
Director's Tel: 503-494-6976

Appendix D: Alzheimer's Disease Research Centers Directory

Director's Fax: 503-494-7499

Pennsylvania

University of Pennsylvania
John Q. Trojanowski, M.D., Ph.D., Director
Alzheimer's Disease Center
Department of Pathology and Laboratory Medicine
University of Pennsylvania School of Medicine
HUP, Maloney 3rd Floor
36th and Spruce Streets
Philadelphia, PA 19104-4283
Website: www.uphs.upenn.edu/ADC
Information Line: 215-662-7810
Director's e-mail: trojanow@mail.med.upenn.edu
Director's Tel: 215-662-4708
Director's Fax: 215-349-5909

University of Pittsburgh
Steven T. DeKosky, M.D., Director
Alzheimer's Disease Research Center
University of Pittsburgh
Department of Neurology
3471 Fifth Avenue, Ste. 811
Pittsburgh, PA 15213-2582
Website: www.adrc.pitt.edu
Information Line: 412-692-2700
Director's e-mail: dekoskyst@upmc.edu
Center's Fax: 412-692-2710

Texas

University of Texas, Southwestern Medical Center
Roger N. Rosenberg, M.D., Director
Alzheimer's Disease Research Center
Department of Neurology
University of Texas SW Medical Center
5323 Harry Hines Boulevard
Dallas, TX 75390-9036
Website: www.utsouthwestern.edu/alzheimers/research
Information Line: 214-648-9394
Director's e-mail: roger.rosenberg@UTsouthwestern.edu

Director's Tel: 214-648-3239
Fax: 214-648-6824

Washington

University of Washington
Murray Raskind, M.D., Director
Alzheimer's Disease Center
VA Puget Sound Health Care System
Mental Health Services, S-116
1660 South Columbian Way
Seattle, WA 98108
Website: http://depts.washington.edu/adrcweb
Information Line: 206-277-3281
Director's e-mail: murray.raskind@med.va.gov
Fax: 206-768-5456

Alzheimer's Disease Cooperative Study (ADCS)

The ADCS conducts clinical trials on promising compounds designed to improve cognitive functioning, slow the rate of decline, or delay the onset of Alzheimer's disease.

University of California, San Diego
9500 Gilman Drive - 0949
La Jolla, CA 92093-0949
Website: http://adcs.ucsd.edu
Information Line: 858-622-5880

Alzheimer's Disease Education and Referral Center

The Center provides information, free publications, and referrals.
PO Box 8259
Silver Spring, MD 20907-8250
Website: www.nia.nih.gov/Alzheimers
Information Line: 1-800-438-4380 (toll free)
E-mail: adear@nia.nih.gov
Fax: 301-495-3334

National Alzheimer's Coordinating Center

The Center coordinates data collection and fosters collaborative research among ADCs.
Walter Kukull, Ph.D., Director
National Alzheimer's Coordinating Center

Appendix D: Alzheimer's Disease Research Centers Directory

4311 11th Avenue NE, #300
Seattle, WA 98105
Website: www.alz.washington.edu
Information Line: 206-543-8637
E-mail: naccmail@u.washington.edu
Fax: 206-616-5927

National Cell Repository for Alzheimer's Disease

The Repository maintains a database of family histories and medical records and provides genetic researchers with cell lines and/or DNA samples.
Tatiana Foroud, Ph.D., Director
Indiana University Medical Center
Department of Medical and Molecular Genetics
975 West Walnut Street, Room IB-130
Indianapolis IN 46202-5251
Website: www.ncrad.org
Information Line: 1-800-526-2839 (toll free)
E-mail: alzstudy@iupui.edu
Fax: 317-274-2387

Appendix E: Why Patients Choose The Mayo Clinic

The reason why half a million people from around the world choose The Mayo Clinic for their medical care each year are:

- Top doctors

    The Mayo Clinic chooses doctors carefully based on their educational background, their medical skills, and their ability to work together. Because of the large volume of patients who come to Mayo for care, doctors quickly gain extensive experience in treating every kind of illness. Many become international experts. The Mayo system supports doctors by making it easy for them to work together and by providing the best personnel, facilities and technology to help them deliver the best care to every patient every day.

- Pioneer in new treatments

    A part of Mayo's mission is to continually look for new and better ways of doing things. Mayo patients are frequently among the first to benefit from new ideas pioneered by Mayo doctors and researchers. The emphasis on learning is what makes Mayo one of the leading centers for educating other doctors.

- Reputation

    Mayo has earned a reputation for solving hard-to-solve medical problems based on more than 100 years of results. This is affirmed by the fact that more than 70 percent of Mayo's patients have previously been seen at Mayo.

- Many viewpoints

    Mayo's system is built on working together, encouraging doctors to freely consult with each other about patients. This is why Mayo doctors are called "consultants." Patients do not get just one opinion at Mayo; they get multiple opinions. The principle at Mayo is two heads are better than one and five are even better.

- Single Location Quality, Efficient & Superior Medical Care

    Virtually all medical services a patient might need -- doctor visits, testing, surgery and hospital care -- are available "under one roof" at The Mayo Clinic. The scheduling of these services is done in a coordinated and efficient way, so that what might take months to accomplish in a community setting can be done in a matter of days at Mayo.

I also believe The Mayo Clinic is one of the few medical institutions in the world that truly practices integrative complementary medicine. What this means is initially you meet with an internal medicine specialist who reviews and further documents your medical history, performs a physical examination and schedules initial tests. If a problem is identified, the internal medicine specialist begins to build a team of doctors who specialize in treating the condition detected. The internal medicine specialist may give a handoff to another specialist, i.e. cardiologist, cancer specialist, neurology who all work together in a complementary manner to treat the problem. This method of treatment is unique to The Mayo Clinic. At other hospitals you deal with a collection of individuals who do not share the same common data and who work as individuals instead of a team. Also, many Mayo Clinic doctors work on a fixed salary so there is no incentive to recommend tests or medications that are not necessary. Outside of The Mayo Clinic, many of the imaging, x-ray and rehabilitation facilities around the country have doctors as their principal investors. Finally, after each visit a complete set of documentation is presented to the patient including lab results and doctors notes so the patient may truly manage their health care. This data then becomes part of a patients long term records at The Mayo Clinic. At many other institutions, the patient has better maintenance and performance information on their motor vehicles than their own health.

Appendix F: Olive's Clinical Diagnosis

Copy

Mayo Clinic
200 First Street SW
Rochester, Minnesota 55905
507-284-2511

Vesna D. Garovic, M.D.
Division of Hypertension
Department of Internal Medicine

January 28, 2002

Mrs. Olive M. Bublitz
217 West Page Street
Elkhorn, WI 53121-1215

RE: Mrs. Olive Mae Bublitz
MC#: 5-059-482
DOB: 1920-8-5

Dear Mrs. Bublitz:

I had the opportunity of seeing you for a medical evaluation in the Division of Hypertension.

Your final diagnoses were:

• Hypertension
• Atrial fibrillation
• Hypertrophic cardiomyopathy
• Decreased hearing
• Degenerative joint disease
• Osteoporosis
• Cognitive impairment

Attached is the clinical documentation which summarizes our impressions and recommendations (Vesna D. Garovic, M.D.: Jan-24-2002, Jan-21-2002; Carroll F. Poppen: Jan-24-2002; Matthew J. Taylor, M.D.: Jan-24-2002; David S. Knopman, M.D.: Jan-23-2002; Mary M. Gallenberg, M.D.: Jan-22-2002). I have also included the most recent laboratory results report.

We are grateful to have the opportunity to participate in your care.

Sincerely,

[signature]

Vesna D. Garovic, M.D.

VDG:bfl
Enclosures

cc: Enclosed is a copy for your local physician.

Appendix F: Olive's Clinical Diagnosis

Jan-24-2002 -Subsequent Visit, Vesna D. Garovic, M.D.,Hypertension

CHIEF COMPLAINT/PURPOSE OF VISIT:
Follow-up appointment.

IMPRESSION/REPORT/PLAN:
I am reviewing lab and test results and consultations with Mrs. Bublitz and her son. I have noted that her CBC was normal, chemistries were acceptable, and her TSH was within the normal range. Her urinalysis was negative and EKG showed a sinus rhythm with a voltage criteria for LVH and rate of 61. This was consistent with her six-hour blood pressure monitoring that showed inadequate blood pressure control of average systolic of 169 and average diastolic of 80. We spoke about these blood pressure readings. I think that we should increase her Lotensin to 40 mg daily. For now, she will start taking two of her 20 mg pills daily. Her son suggested that she is planning to get a home blood pressure device and to monitor her blood pressure. If her blood pressure does not come down to 140/90 on an increased dose of Lotensin, the next step would be to add a low dose of diuretic such as hydrochlorothiazide 12.5 mg to her daily regimen.
I noted that Mrs. Bublitz was seen by a neurologist. They suggested lumbar puncture but she decided to defer that at present. She will be leaving for Los Angeles with her son and he is planning to have her enrolled in a daily social activity in a local adult center.
I noted that she was seen by a gynecologist and had a normal Pap smear. They also requested a densitometry bone scan that showed established osteoporosis. I suggested that Mrs. Bublitz needs to be followed up by a physician when she moves to L.A. and some form of treatment including hormone replacement therapy should be considered. I have given her my card in the case that they have any other issues or questions for me. Mrs. Bublitz also had an ear, nose, and throat evaluation and removal of wax from her right ear.

DIAGNOSES:
#1 Hypertension
#2 Atrial fibrillation
#3 Hypertrophic cardiomyopathy
#4 Decreased hearing
#5 Degenerative joint disease
#6 Osteoporosis
#7 Cognitive impairment

VDG:bfl Revised: Jan-25-2002 09:12

Jan-24-2002 -Consult, Carroll F. Poppen,Otorhinolaryngology

REFERRAL:
Dr. Vesna D. Garovic (4-7979).

CHIEF COMPLAINT/PURPOSE OF VISIT:
Hearing loss.

HISTORY OF PRESENT ILLNESS:
Mrs. Bublitz is an 81-year-old white female who presents with her son for ear, nose, and throat consultation. She has a past history of a hearing loss, more so on her left ear than right ear, which has been present for a number of years. She mostly does pretty well with one-on-one communication. Her family members have noticed that she has had some hearing loss. She denies any tinnitus or vertigo. She denies any ear pain, redness, swelling, or discharge. She has a past history of chronic ear disease as a child. She has no other ear, nose, and throat problems.

PHYSICAL EXAMINATION:
ENT:

This is a printout from the electronic medical record and is the most current version as of the date and time printed.

Ears: Right canal was clear. Right tympanic membrane is scarred. There was a dry, hard plug of wax in the left ear canal in the attic area which was removed. She does have some marked amount of scarring on the left tympanic membrane. There is also some whitish discoloration up above which may possibly represent tympanosclerosis or perhaps a cholesteatoma.
Nose: Normal.
Oropharynx: Normal.
Audiogram reveals a left mixed loss and a right sensorineural loss.

IMPRESSION/REPORT/PLAN:
#1 History of chronic ear disease, rule out cholesteatoma
  RECOMMENDATIONS
  Consultation with Dr. Matthew J. Taylor of our department to examine her right ear to rule out any other possible middle ear disease.

DIAGNOSES:
#1 History of chronic ear disease, rule out cholesteatoma

CFP:nlb

Jan-24-2002 -Consult, Matthew J. Taylor, M.D.,Otorhinolaryngology

REFERRAL:
Mr. Carroll Poppen

CHIEF COMPLAINT/PURPOSE OF VISIT:
Rule-out cholesteatoma on the left ear.

HISTORY OF PRESENT ILLNESS:
Mrs. Bublitz is a very pleasant 81-year-old female who has had difficulty with hearing on the left side for several years. Ever since she was a child, she remembers having problems with recurrent ear infections. She does not recall having ear surgery in the past, but she does recall being taken to the ear doctor on several occasions to have the ear cleaned.

PHYSICAL EXAMINATION:
General: She is an alert, well-nourished female in no acute distress.
Eyes: Extraocular movements are intact. Pupils are equal, round, and reactive to light. No periorbital erythema or edema.
ENT:
  Ears: She was taken to the Otomicroscope Room. The right external auditory canal and ear and appears within normal limits. The left ear external canal is within normal limits. She has a monomeric appearing drum that is retracted down to the promontory; however, there is absence of a malleus. I do see that the eardrum is draped over the body of the incus. There is no retraction pocket or squamous debris present. I was able to palpate the whitish area in the superior region of the middle ear and palpated it as bone and not cholesteatoma.

IMPRESSION/REPORT/PLAN:
#1 Left conductive hearing loss secondary to ossicular disruption
  It appears that this has been operated on in the past. Certainly the physical exam findings would explain her conductive hearing loss. She would certainly benefit from a hearing aid on that side, but she is not interested in pursuing this at this time. She should have her hearing checked and a re-examination done in one year. All questions were answered.

DIAGNOSES:
#1 Left conductive hearing loss secondary to ossicular disruption

This is a printout from the electronic medical record and is the most current version as of the date and time printed.

Appendix F: Olive's Clinical Diagnosis

MJT:rmb

Jan-23-2002 -Consult, David S. Knopman, M.D.,Neurology

REFERRAL:
Doctor Garovic-Kocic 47979

CHIEF COMPLAINT/PURPOSE OF VISIT:
Confusion

HISTORY OF PRESENT ILLNESS:
Mrs. Bublitz is an 81-year-old woman who is accompanied by her son. Mrs. Bublitz was involved in a minor motor vehicle accident in November near Thanksgiving and immediately thereafter her son said that she has been confused. He feels that the confusion has been stable since that point but hasn't improved at all. He had been with her prior to the accident for about three months up until November 12. Over that time, he noted that his mother had some mild forgetfulness such as walking into a room and not knowing why she went in there but he felt that she was otherwise independent at that time in her activities of daily living. Mrs. Bublitz lives by herself in Elkhorn, Wisconsin and had been driving, managing all of her affairs and generally taking care of herself quite well. Her son had been with her for those three months because she had a number of health problems and had been back and forth to the Mayo Clinic because of her cardiac issues.

Since the accident, she's had problems with orientation for time and she's had significant short term memory loss. She's been unable to manage her checkbook. In addition, her son noticed that her walking has been abnormal and that she takes short stride, seems unsteady and has difficulty turning quickly without losing her balance. He also noted that a longstanding problem of urinary urgency has gotten worse. The patient herself has some insight into these issues but it is probably incomplete. She spontaneously gave up driving. She says that she remembers the motor vehicle accident quite clearly. She did not lose consciousness. She was taken home immediately after the accident by a law enforcement officer and she remembers that.

The patient has significant heart disease in the form of atrial fibrillation and cardiomyopathy. She is not on Coumadin. There have been no changes in her medications.

REVIEWED PMH, ALLERGIES, SH, FH, MEDICATIONS, AND ROS AS NOTED ON THE CURRENT VISIT INFORMATION FORM, DATED 18-SEP-2001 AND ON THE PATIENT FAMILY HISTORY FORM DATED 18-SEP-2001, PERTINENT INFORMATION INCLUDES:

CURRENT MEDICATIONS:
Lotensin 20 mg daily
diltiazem CD 120 mg daily
amiodarone 200 mg daily
aspirin 81 mg daily
vitamin C 500 mg daily
vitamin E 400 IU daily
multivitamin daily
milk of magnesia daily

ALLERGIES:
Penicillin

SYSTEMS REVIEW:
Mild visual difficulties, dizziness, constipation, low back pain, tenderness over her occipital region.

PAST MEDICAL/SURGICAL HISTORY
1. Hypertension.

This is a printout from the electronic medical record and is the most current version as of the date and time printed.

2. Atrial fibrillation.
3. Hypertrophic cardiomyopathy.
4. Cataracts.
5. Decreased hearing.
6. Degenerative joint disease.

SOCIAL HISTORY:
Patient lives by herself
She doesn't use tobacco or alcohol products

FAMILY HISTORY:
Not contributory
See PFH

PHYSICAL EXAMINATION:
Neuro: Please see the neuro exam sheet dated 1/23/02. On mental status examination, Mrs. Bublitz thought the
year was 2001 and she was unable to recall any of four words after five minutes. She had great difficulty
with constructions and calculations while fund of knowledge was intact. She denied being depressed but she
admitted to being lonely and frustrated by her problems. Note that since she hasn't been driving, she's been
by herself in her home without much company.

On the remainder of her neurologic exam, her facies had a slight reduction in mobility but extraocular
movements and visual fields were full. Reflexes were brisk throughout and I thought that her right toe was
probably up while the left was equivocal. Her balance was impaired in that she could not stand on her heels
or toes nor could she tandem walk. Romberg sign showed some swaying. Otherwise, the remainder of her
motor and sensory exam was unremarkable as was the coordination exam for finger-to-nose maneuver,
heel-to-shin or rapid alternating movements.

I reviewed her MR scan of yesterday. It showed no acute lesions. The amount of white matter change was
minimal. There was prominent cerebral atrophy and ventricular enlargement but she does not have
hydrocephalus. Hippocampal atrophy was quite striking.

Laboratory tests are largely pending but her CBC is normal. Other studies should be back later today which
would be pertinent.

IMPRESSION/REPORT/PLAN:
#1 Cognitive impairment
There is a major conceptual issue here as to whether Mrs. Bublitz is experiencing a subacute dementing
illness of two months duration or whether in fact she has a more longstanding chronic process and this
merely represents a slight exaggeration of an existing condition. I favor the latter. That is, I believe that she
probably had an underlying dementing illness, probably Alzheimer's disease, for some time that was well
compensated. Then with her minor motor vehicle accident, which I believe caused no significant brain
injury, it upset her usual scheme of activities and made her seem more confused and disabled her
compensatory mechanisms. Also, her relative social isolation by not being able to drive may have
exacerbated the problem further. If this hypothesis is correct, then she is unlikely to show any substantial
improvement over time but neither is she likely to worsen dramatically either. This would mean that her
living situation at the present time is probably not satisfactory and she would need to be in a more stable
living situation, probably with her son out where he lives in Los Angeles.

The alternative hypothesis is that she has a more rapidly progressive dementing illness and it could worsen
dramatically. The laboratory studies back so far and the imaging study don't support any such structural or
metabolic cause but there are many pending laboratory studies. Furthering this diagnostic issue, she should
have a lumbar puncture to make sure that she doesn't have a CNS infection, occult cancer, or even less likely
Creutzfeldt-Jakob disease as a cause of her rapidly progressive changes in status. I have ordered a lumbar
puncture and I believe that she will consent to have it done.

This is a printout from the electronic medical record and is the most current version as of the date and
time printed.

Appendix F: Olive's Clinical Diagnosis

Unfortunately, I think it is unlikely that Mrs. Bublitz has a readily reversible condition. I shared this concern with her son though I left the door open for the prospect that she would not change dramatically in the near future.

If timing permits, I'd be happy to see Mrs. Bublitz back but that will probably have to be next week. If there are any questions, please feel free to contact me by the end of the day Thursday.

DIAGNOSES:
#1 Confusional syndrome, dementia versus subacute dementia
#2 Cardiomyopathy
#3 Atrial fibrillation

DSK:vam

Jan-22-2002 -Consult, Mary M. Gallenberg, M.D.,Gynecology

REFERRAL:
Vesna Garovic-Kocic, M.D. (4-7979)

CHIEF COMPLAINT/PURPOSE OF VISIT:
Gynecologic examination

HISTORY OF PRESENT ILLNESS:
Patient is an 81-year-old, gravida 3, para 1, white female seen at the request of Dr. Garovic for GYN examination. Last menstrual period was around age 50. She has never had any postmenopausal bleeding. No hormone replacement therapy. She denies any hot flashes. No vaginal dryness. She is not sexually active. No stress incontinence of urine. No history of GYN surgery. No history of abnormal Papanicolaou smears.

PHYSICAL EXAMINATION:
Abdomen: No palpable masses, tenderness, or organomegaly.
Pelvis: External genitalia normal. Vagina atrophic. Cervix normal. Papanicolaou smear taken (scrape and cytobrush). Uterus small, mobile, nontender. Adnexa no masses or tenderness. Rectovaginal confirms.

IMPRESSION/REPORT/PLAN:
#1 Atrophic vaginitis

Recommendation:
We discussed hormone replacement therapy. The patient is not interested in hormonal therapy. Her son is concerned with her decreasing height. She is 152 cm tall and weighs 119 pounds. I have requested a bone density and she will follow-up with Dr. Garovic for the results.

MMG:kgc
Electronically signed Jan-22-2002 11:34 by M.M. Gallenberg, M.D.

Jan-21-2002 -Multi-system Evaluation, Vesna D. Garovic, M.D.,Hypertension

CHIEF COMPLAINT/PURPOSE OF VISIT:
The patient is an 81-year-old woman from Elkhorn, Wisconsin, with a past medical history of hypertension, atrial fibrillation, and hypertrophic cardiomyopathy who comes to Mayo with complaints of memory difficulties after a car accident in November of last year.

HISTORY OF PRESENT ILLNESS:
The patient has had a history of hypertension for more than 20 years. In addition, she has atrial fibrillation and

This is a printout from the electronic medical record and is the most current version as of the date and time printed.

hypertrophic cardiomyopathy for which she is followed up here at Mayo since 1996. She was last seen in our clinic in September of 2001 for problems with her blood pressure. At that time, she was experiencing constipation on Cardizem, and the dose of that was cut from 240 mg CD to 120 mg CD. In addition, she was prescribed milk of magnesia with good control of her bowel movements. She was doing very well until November of this year when she was involved in a motor vehicle accident. She basically suffered from an injury in the soft tissue of her neck and, ever since, she has been experiencing headaches associated with dizziness increasing the problems with her memory. She did have that in the past but both she and her son, who accompanies her today, think that it is getting worse since the accident. She did not suffer a loss of consciousness. No history of seizure disorder. No lightheadedness. No palpitations or chest pain. No lower extremity swelling. Her health maintenance measures are current in terms of the mammogram that was done in September of 2001 which was negative and colon screening testing done at the same time reported no abnormalities. She had an echocardiogram at that time which showed an ejection fraction of 78% and abnormal left ventricular relaxation. She did not have a gynecology exam and Pap smear for approximately ten years.

REVIEWED PMH, ALLERGIES, SH, FH, MEDICATIONS, AND ROS AS NOTED ON THE CURRENT VISIT INFORMATION FORM, DATED 18-SEP-2001 AND ON THE PATIENT FAMILY HISTORY FORM DATED 18-SEP-2001, PERTINENT INFORMATION INCLUDES:

CURRENT MEDICATIONS:
Lotensin 20 mg daily
diltiazem CD 120 mg daily
amiodarone 200 mg daily
aspirin 81 mg daily
vitamin C 500 mg daily
vitamin E 400 IU daily
multivitamin daily
milk of magnesia daily

ALLERGIES:
penicillin

SYSTEMS REVIEW:
1. Blurred vision due to cataracts.
2. Dizziness.
3. Memory difficulties.
4. Constipation - improved on current regimen.
5. Lower back pain.
6. Sleep apnea

PAST MEDICAL/SURGICAL HISTORY
1. Hypertension.
2. Atrial fibrillation.
3. Hypertrophic cardiomyopathy.
4. Cataracts.
5. Decreased hearing.
6. Degenerative joint disease.

SOCIAL HISTORY:
She does not smoke or drink. Her husband died from a heart attack. She has one son.

PHYSICAL EXAMINATION:
Blood pressure: 180/90, supine/seated (observed Jan-21-2002).
General: Very pleasant elderly frail woman in no acute distress.
Head: Normal.
Eyes: Bilateral cataract. Status post surgery.
ENT: Decreased hearing.

This is a printout from the electronic medical record and is the most current version as of the date and time printed.

Appendix F: Olive's Clinical Diagnosis

Vessels: 3+ and equal bilaterally. No carotid bruit appreciated.
Heart: S1, S2. 1-2/6 systolic murmur.
Lungs: Clear to A&P.
Abdomen: Soft and benign. No organomegaly.
Spine: Nontender.
Joints: Full range of motion.
Extremities: No clubbing, cyanosis, or edema.
Gait: Somewhat unsteady with short steps.

IMPRESSION/REPORT/PLAN:

#1 Hypertension

Her blood pressure is not adequately controlled. Both the patient and her son raised the possibility that she might be anxious having to undergo an MRI and that this might be resulting in her elevated blood pressures today. To further evaluate this, we are going to obtain a six-hour blood pressure monitoring. We will obtain chemistries including kidney function tests, liver function tests, UA, ECG, and chest x-ray.

#2 Memory problems

This seems to have become worse after the motor vehicle accident. To evaluate this further, we are going to schedule her for an MRI of the head and neck and MRA of the cerebral vasculature. We will also schedule her to see Neurology. Prior to that, we are going to obtain baseline chemistries including B12 and folate levels.

#3 Atrial fibrillation - stable on current medications

She is going to continue on the current medications.

#4 Health maintenance

Her mammogram and colon screening testing is up to date. We will send her to see a gynecologist as she did not have a gynecologic exam for approximately ten years. We will also check her lipid profile. We will check the TSH, especially in the setting of memory problems.

VDG:slj

```
05059482 BUBLITZ, Olive                    Mayo Clinic Results Summary          Page 1 (more)
Run Date/Time: 28Jan2002  9:06am                                                Report ID: ALL REPORTS & LABS
Reporting period = 30Oct2001 thru 28Jan2002  Requested by: MRG0351
```

```
Age in years      : 81          Date of Birth   : 1920-08-05        Gender      : F
Location          :
```

LABORATORY

```
LAB AG
                                           23Jan2002
HEMATOLOGY AG         Reference Range          07:29
  HEMATOLOGY I AG                              ROCH
  Hemoglobin...........12.0-15.5   g/dL        13.9
  Hematocrit...........34.9-44.5   %           41.4
  Erythrocytes.........3.90-5.03   x10(12)/L   4.58
  MCV..................81.6-98.3   fL          90.4
  RBC Distrib Width....11.9-15.5   %           13.7
  Leukocytes...........3.5-10.5    x10(9)/L    8.1
  Neutrophils..........1.7-7.0     x10(9)/L    5.32
  Monocytes............0.3-0.9     x10(9)/L    0.80
  Lymphocytes..........0.9-2.9     x10(9)/L    1.61
  Basophils............0-0.3       x10(9)/L    0.02
  Eosinophils..........0.05-0.50   x10(9)/L    0.30
  Platelet Count.......150-450     x10(9)/L    208
  MPV..................7.4-10.9     fL          7.9
====================================================================================================
                                           23Jan2002
SPECIAL HEMATOLOGY AG Reference Range          07:29
  B-12/FOLATE/IRON GRP AG                      ROCH
  B-12 Assay(S)........200-650     ng/L        257
  Folate(S)............>= 3.5      ug/L        13.8
====================================================================================================
                                           23Jan2002
CHEMISTRY AG          Reference Range          07:29
  BLOOD CHEMISTRY 1 AG                         ROCH
  Sodium...............135-145     mEq/L       146   *
  Potassium............3.6-4.8     mEq/L       4.0
  Calcium..............8.9-10.1    mg/dL       9.1
  Glucose(P)...........70-100      mg/dL       96
  Alk Phosphatase......119-309     U/L         188
  AST (GOT)............12-31       U/L         16
====================================================================================================
                                           23Jan2002
CHEMISTRY AG          Reference Range          07:29
  BLOOD CHEMISTRY 2 AG                         ROCH
  Creatinine...........0.6-0.9     mg/dL       1.0   *
====================================================================================================
                                           23Jan2002
CHEMISTRY AG          Reference Range          07:29
  CARDIAC CHEMISTRY AG                         ROCH
  LDH (S)........8344 R112-257     U/L         157
====================================================================================================
                                           23Jan2002
ENZYMES AG            Reference Range          07:29
  ENZYMES I AG                                 ROCH
  ALT (GPT)(S).........9-29        U/L         13
====================================================================================================
                                           23Jan2002
ENDOCRINE AG          Reference Range          07:29
  ENDOCRINE I AG                               ROCH
  Sensitive TSH(S)......0.30-5.0   mIU/L       2.1
====================================================================================================
                                           22Jan2002
Urinalysis Tests AG   Reference Range          08:58
  URINALYSIS, ROUTINE AG                       ROCH
  Source...................                    VOID
  Appearance...........Normal                  Normal
  Osmolality...........300-800     mosm/Kg     633
  pH.......................                    7.9
  Glucose..............<25         mg/dL       3
  Protein..............         mg/dL          4
  Protein/Osmoloality...<0.12      Ratio       0.06
  Predicted 24h Protein.          mg/24 h      54
  Predicted Range.......          mg/24 h      13-221
====================================================================================================
                                           23Jan2002
Urinalysis Tests AG   Reference Range          08:58
```

Appendix F: Olive's Clinical Diagnosis

05059482 BUBLITZ, Olive
Run Date/Time: 28Jan2002 9:06am
Reporting period = 30Oct2001 thru 28Jan2002 Requested by: MRG0351

Mayo Clinic Results Summary

Page 2 (more)
Report ID: ALL REPORTS & LABS

```
                                        22Jan2002
Urinalysis Tests AG   Reference Range      08:58
  URINE MICROSCOPY AG                       ROCH
Microscopy...........Normal               ABNORM*
  RBC.................Occ <1      /hpf     Occ <1
  WBC.................1-3         /hpf     4-10  *
  Casts,Hyaline.......            /lpf     OCCAS
```

ECG

ECG Reports

```
21Jan2002 13:50
VENTRICULAR RATE 61
Normal sinus rhythm with 1st degree A-V block
Moderate voltage criteria for LVH, may be normal
variant
Nonspecific ST and T wave abnormality
When compared with ECG of 19-SEP-2001 11:45,
No significant change was found
47857^OLNEY  MD^BYRON
```

MICROBIOLOGY

Microbiology by Specimen Source
No Matching Data Found

RADIOLOGY

Radiology Reports

```
23Jan2002 11:24AM  Exam: NM Bone Density Spine & Hip
    Indications: MEASURE BONE MINERAL CONTENT
    01/23/2002 11:58AM   RMH
    Lumbar Spine:
    L2: BMD = 0.84 g/cm(sq), T Score = -3.0, Z Score = -0.6
    TOTAL BMD = 0.84 g/cm(sq),  (27th percentile)
    T Score = -3.0      Z Score = -0.6
    Osteoporosis is established when the T Score is below -2.50.
    NONDIAGNOSTIC SPINE DUE TO DEGENERATIVE CHANGES.  RECOMMEND
    HIP ONLY FOR FUTURE FOLLOWUP.
    Left Hip:
    FEMUR NECK: BMD = 0.62 g/cm (sq)  (27th percentile)
    T Score = -3.0      Z Score = -0.6
    Osteoporosis is established when the T Score is below -2.50.
    Additional FEMUR measurements listed below:
    TROCH: BMD = 0.49 g/cm(sq)  (18th percentile)
    T Score = -2.7      Z Score = -0.9
    INTER: BMD = 0.72 g/cm(sq)
    WARD'S: BMD = 0.43 g/cm(sq)  (21st percentile)
    T Score = -3.7      Z Score = -0.8
    TOTAL BMD = 0.63 g/cm(sq),  (31st percentile)
    T Score = -3.0      Z Score = -0.5
    ** ELECTRONIC IMAGES ONLY
    L.A. Forstrom  4-7361


22Jan2002 2:32PM  Exam: MRI & MRA HEAD W/O
22Jan2002 2:33PM  Exam: MRI CERVICAL SPINE
    Indications: MRI/MRA Head/Brain MRI^Cervical spine, sedation;
    memory change and soft tissue cervical trauma; s/p mva
    Indications: MRI/MRA Head/Brain MRI^Cervical spine, sedation
    01/22/2002   3:13PM   RMH
    MR examination of the cervical spine, as well as MR
    examination of the head, including intracranial MR angiogram
    performed.
    The cervical study demonstrates generalized degenerative disk
    disease throughout the mid and lower cervical spine with disk
```

05059482 BUBLITZ, Olive
Run Date/Time: 28Jan2002 9:06am
Reporting period = 30Oct2001 thru 28Jan2002 Requested by: MRG0351

Mayo Clinic Results Summary

Page 3 (more)
Report ID:ALL REPORTS & LABS

22Jan2002 2:32PM Exam: MRI & MRA HEAD W/O (Continued)

    space narrowing and generalized disk bulging at multiple
levels. There is mild central canal narrowing at the C4-5 and
C5-6 levels, though the cervical spinal cord is normal.
Examination of the head demontrates moderate generalized
cerebral and mild generalized cerebellar atrophy. There are a
few scattered focal areas of signal abnormality in the white
matter of both cerebral hemispheres, likely representing small
vessel degenerative change. The intracranial angiogram is
normal.
(C) (RVU202)
M. J. Kiely MD. 4-7844

21Jan2002 3:03PM Exam: Chest-- PA & Lateral
    Indications: atrial fibrillation
01/21/2002 3:58PM ROMAYO
Cardiomegaly. Pulmonary venous hypertension. Mitral annulus
calcification. Calcified mediastinal lymph nodes.
(RVU104)
J. Gurney, M.D. 4-7691

PATHOLOGY

Pathology Reports

22Jan2002 Cytology Gynecological
Requested By: Vesna Garovic, M.D.
(PR02-7129)
    DIAGNOSIS:
       Cervical/Endocervical Smear
       Satisfactory for evaluation but limited by.
         No Endocervical Cells Identified.
       Within Normal Limits.
    23Jan2002   Michael R. Christensen, CT(ASCP)
    23Jan2002   GLK 46160:mrc

AUTONOMIC

Autonomic Lab Reports
No Matching Data Found

EEG

EEG Reports
No Matching Data Found

EMG

EMG Reports
No Matching Data Found

MOVEMENT DISORDERS

Movement Disorders Reports
No Matching Data Found

CATH

Cath Reports
No Matching Data Found

ECHO

ECHO Reports
No Matching Data Found

Appendix F: Olive's Clinical Diagnosis

05059482 BUBLITZ, Olive
Run Date/Time: 28Jan2002 9:06am
Reporting period = 30Oct2001 thru 28Jan2002 Requested by: MRG0351

Mayo Clinic Results Summary

Page 4 (last)
Report ID: ALL REPORTS & LABS

	SURGERY

Surgical Reports
No Matching Data Found

	TRANSFUSION MEDICINE

Tx Med Reports
No Matching Data Found

	PENDING RESULTS

Pending Results
No Pending Data Found

	LEGENDS

ROCH   = L. E. Wold, M.D.   ,Laboratory Director
ROCHESTER   200 SW First Street   Rochester   MN 55905

*** End of data ***
No data errors detected

Appendix G: Extended Hospice Patient Re-qualification

WORKSHEET TO DETERMINE PROGNOSIS

DEMENTIA

Dementia due to Alzheimer's Disease and Related Disorders

Patients will be considered to be in the terminal stage of dementia (life expectancy of six months or less) if they meet the following criteria.

Patients with dementia should show all the following characteristics:
_____ a. Stage seven or beyond according to the Functional assessment Staging Scale.
_____ b. Unable to ambulate without assist. _____ c. Unable to dress without assist.
_____ d. Unable to bathe without assist. _____ e. Urinary and fecal incontinence
(intermittent or constant)
_____ f. No consistently meaningful verbal communication: stereotypical phrases only, or the ability to speak is limited to six or fewer intelligible words.

Patient should have had one of the following within the past 12 months:
_____ a. Aspiration pneumonia _____ b. Pyelonephritis or upper urinary tract infection.
_____ c. Septicemia _____ d. Decubitus ulcers, multiple, stages 3-4
_____ e. Fever recurrent after antibiotics
_____ f. Inability to maintain sufficient fluid and calorie intake with 10% weight loss during the previous six months or serum albumin less than 2.5 gm/dl

Note: This section is specific for Alzheimer's Disease and Related Disorders, and not appropriate for other types of dementia.

CO-MORBIDITIES: KPS or PPS must be <70%
_____ KPS SCORE OR _____ PPS SCORE

Appendix G: Extended Hospice Patient Re-qualification

FUNCTIONAL ASSESSMENT STAGING (FAST) FOR DEMENTIA

Stage	Based on information from knowledgeable source
1	No difficulties, either subjectively or objectively.
2	Complains of forgetting location of objects; subjective word finding difficulties only.
3	Decreased job functioning evident to coworkers; difficulty in traveling to new locations.
4	Decreased ability to perform complex tasks (e.g., planning dinner for guests; handling finances; marketing).
5	Requires assistance in choosing proper clothing for the season or occasion.
6a	Difficulty putting clothing on properly without assistance.
6b	Unable to bathe properly; may develop fear of bathing. Will usually require assistance adjusting bath water temperature.
6c	Inability to handle mechanics of toileting (i.e., forgets to flush; doesn't wipe properly).
6d	Urinary incontinence, occasional or more frequent.
6e	Fecal incontinence, occasional or more frequent.
7a	Ability to speak limited to about half a dozen words in an average day.
7b	Intelligible vocabulary limited to a single word in an average day.
7c	Nonambulatory (unable to walk without assistance).
7d	Unable to sit up independently.
7e	Unable to smile.
7f	Unable to hold head up.

KARNOFSKY PERFORMANCE STATUS SCALE DEFINITIONS RATING (%) CRITERIA

Able to carry on normal activity and to work; no special care needed.	100	Normal no complaints; no evidence of disease.
	90	Able to carry on normal activity; minor signs or symptoms of disease.
	80	Normal activity with effort; some signs or symptoms of disease.
Unable to work; able to live at home and care for most personal needs; varying amount of assistance needed.	70	Cares for self; unable to carry on normal activity or to do active work.
	60	Requires occasional assistance, but is able to care for most of his personal needs.
	50	Requires considerable assistance and frequent medical care.
Unable to care for self; requires equivalent of institutional or hospital care; disease may be progressing rapidly.	40	Disabled; requires special care and assistance.
	30	Severely disabled; hospital admission is indicated although death not imminent.
	20	Very sick; hospital admission necessary; active supportive treatment necessary.
	10	Moribund; fatal processes progressing rapidly.
	0	Dead

PALLIATIVE PERFORMANCE SCALE (PPS)

Ambulation	Activity & Evidence of Disease	Self-Care	Intake	Conscious Level	Percent
Full	Normal, none	Full	Normal	Full	100
Full	Normal, some evidence	Full	Normal	Full	90
Full	Normal with effort, some evidence	Full	Normal or reduced	Full	80
Reduced	Unable to perform normal job or work, some evidence	Full	Normal or reduced	Full	70
Reduced	Unable to do a hobby or work around home, significant disease evidence	Occasional assistance necessary	Normal or reduced	Full or confusion	60
Mainly sit or lie	Unable to do any work, extensive disease	Considerable assistance required	Normal or reduced	Full or confusion	50
Mainly in bed	Unable to do any work, extensive disease	Mainly assistance	Normal or reduced	Full or drowsy or confusion	40
Totally bed bound	Unable to do any work. Extensive disease	Total care	Reduced	Full or drowsy or confusion	30
Totally bed bound	Unable to do any work, extensive disease	Total care	Minimal sips	Full or drowsy or confusion	20
Totally bed bound	Unable to do any work, extensive disease	Total care	Mouth care only	Drowsy or coma	10
Dead	NA	NA	NA	NA	0

Appendix H: Olive's Certificate of Death

CERTIFICATE OF DEATH
STATE OF CALIFORNIA
USE BLACK INK ONLY / NO ERASURES, WHITEOUTS OR ALTERATIONS
VS-11 (REV 1/96)

1. NAME OF DECEDENT — FIRST (Given)	2. MIDDLE	3. LAST (Family)
OLIVE	MAE	BUBLITZ

AKA, ALSO KNOWN AS — Include full AKA (FIRST, MIDDLE, LAST)	4. DATE OF BIRTH mm/dd/ccyy	5. AGE Yrs.	IF UNDER ONE YEAR — Months / Days	IF UNDER 24 HOURS — Hours / Minutes	6. SEX
--	08/05/1920	87			F

9. BIRTH STATE/FOREIGN COUNTRY	10. SOCIAL SECURITY NUMBER	11. EVER IN U.S. ARMED FORCES?	12. MARITAL STATUS (at Time of Death)	7. DATE OF DEATH mm/dd/ccyy	9. HOUR (24 Hours)
WISCONSIN	390-16-7457	YES [X] NO [ ] UNK	WIDOWED	08/15/2007	2245

13. EDUCATION — Higher Level/Degree (see worksheet on back)	14/15. WAS DECEDENT HISPANIC/LATINO(A)/SPANISH? (If yes, see worksheet on back)	16. DECEDENT'S RACE — Up to 3 races may be listed (see worksheet on back)
HS GRADUATE	[ ] YES [X] NO	WHITE

17. USUAL OCCUPATION — Type of work for most of life. DO NOT USE RETIRED	18. KIND OF BUSINESS OR INDUSTRY (e.g., grocery store, road construction, employment agency, etc.)	19. YEARS IN OCCUPATION
BOOKKEEPER	MUSICAL INSTRUMENT MANUFACTURING	30

20. DECEDENT'S RESIDENCE (Street and number or location)
4400 SEVENOAKS COURT

21. CITY	22. COUNTY/PROVINCE	23. ZIP CODE	24. YEARS IN COUNTY	25. STATE/FOREIGN COUNTRY
WESTLAKE VILLAGE	LOS ANGELES	91361	6	CALIFORNIA

26. INFORMANT'S NAME, RELATIONSHIP	27. INFORMANT'S MAILING ADDRESS (Street and number or rural route number, city or town, state, ZIP)
ROBERT BUBLITZ, SON	4400 SEVENOAKS CT., WESTLAKE VILLAGE, CA 91361

28. NAME OF SURVIVING SPOUSE — FIRST	29. MIDDLE	30. LAST (Maiden Name)
--	--	--

31. NAME OF FATHER — FIRST	32. MIDDLE	33. LAST	34. BIRTH STATE
JOSEPH	--	SKOTZKE	POLAND

35. NAME OF MOTHER — FIRST	36. MIDDLE	37. LAST (Maiden)	38. BIRTH STATE
EVELYN	--	ALBRIGHT	WI

39. DISPOSITION DATE mm/dd/ccyy	40. PLACE OF FINAL DISPOSITION
08/21/2007	ROSELAWN MEMORIAL GARDENS, 3045 STATE RD. 67, LAKE GENEVA, WI 53147

41. TYPE OF DISPOSITION(S)	42. SIGNATURE OF EMBALMER	43. LICENSE NUMBER
TR/BU	Antonio Carino	9024

44. NAME OF FUNERAL ESTABLISHMENT	45. LICENSE NUMBER	46. SIGNATURE OF LOCAL REGISTRAR	47. DATE mm/dd/ccyy
REARDON SIMI VALLEY FUNERAL HOME	FD 1091		08/20/2007

101. PLACE OF DEATH	102. IF HOSPITAL, SPECIFY ONE	103. IF OTHER THAN HOSPITAL, SPECIFY ONE
LEISURE LIVING	IP [ ] ER/OP [ ] DOA [ ]	Hospice [ ] Nursing Home/LTC [ ] Decedent's Home [ ] Other [X]

104. COUNTY	105. FACILITY ADDRESS OR LOCATION WHERE FOUND (Street and number or location)	106. CITY
LOS ANGELES	29322 DEEP SHADOW DRIVE	AGOURA HILLS

107. CAUSE OF DEATH	Enter the chain of events — diseases, injuries, or complications — that directly caused death. DO NOT enter terminal events such as cardiac arrest, respiratory arrest, or ventricular fibrillation without showing the etiology. DO NOT ABBREVIATE.	Time Interval Between Onset and Death	108. DEATH REPORTED TO CORONER?
IMMEDIATE CAUSE (A) (Final disease or condition resulting in death)	ALZHEIMER'S DEMENTIA	(A?) YEARS	YES [ ] NO [X] REFERRAL NUMBER
Sequentially list conditions, if any, leading to cause on Line A. Enter UNDERLYING CAUSE (disease or injury that initiated the events resulting in death) LAST (B)		(BT)	109. BIOPSY PERFORMED? YES [ ] NO [X]
(C)		(CT)	110. AUTOPSY PERFORMED? YES [ ] NO [X]
(D)		(DT)	111. USED IN DETERMINING CAUSE? YES [ ] NO [X]

112. OTHER SIGNIFICANT CONDITIONS CONTRIBUTING TO DEATH BUT NOT RESULTING IN THE UNDERLYING CAUSE GIVEN IN 107
NONE

113. WAS OPERATION PERFORMED FOR ANY CONDITION IN ITEM 107 OR 112? (If yes, list type of operation and date.)	113A. IF FEMALE, PREGNANT IN LAST YEAR?
NO	YES [ ] NO [X] UNK [ ]

114. I CERTIFY THAT TO THE BEST OF MY KNOWLEDGE DEATH OCCURRED AT THE HOUR, DATE, AND PLACE STATED FROM THE CAUSES STATED.	115. SIGNATURE AND TITLE OF CERTIFIER	116. LICENSE NUMBER	117. DATE mm/dd/ccyy
Decedent Attended Since (A) mm/dd/ccyy 05/12/2006 / Decedent Last Seen Alive (B) mm/dd/ccyy 08/14/2007	Razmig Krumian	20A7776	08/17/2007
	118. TYPE ATTENDING PHYSICIAN'S NAME, MAILING ADDRESS, ZIP CODE: RAZMIG KRUMIAN, D.O., 32144 AGOURA ROAD, SUITE 218 WESTLAKE VILLAGE, CA 91361		

119. I CERTIFY THAT IN MY OPINION DEATH OCCURRED AT THE HOUR, DATE, AND PLACE STATED FROM THE CAUSES STATED.	120. INJURED AT WORK?	121. INJURY DATE mm/dd/ccyy	122. HOUR (24 Hours)
MANNER OF DEATH: Natural [ ] Accident [ ] Homicide [ ] Suicide [ ] Pending Investigation [ ] Could not be determined [ ]	YES [ ] NO [ ] UNK [ ]		

123. PLACE OF INJURY (e.g., home, construction site, wooded area, etc.)

124. DESCRIBE HOW INJURY OCCURRED (Events which resulted in injury)
COPY

125. LOCATION OF INJURY (Street and number, or location, and city, and ZIP)

126. SIGNATURE OF CORONER / DEPUTY CORONER	127. DATE mm/dd/ccyy	128. TYPE NAME, TITLE OF CORONER / DEPUTY CORONER

STATE REGISTRAR	A	B	C	D	E	FAX AUTH. #	CENSUS TRACT
						197/8916	

Appendix I: Olive's Autopsy Results

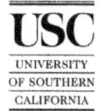

UNIVERSITY OF SOUTHERN CALIFORNIA

Keck School of Medicine
University of Southern California

January 14, 2008

Memory and Aging Center

NIH Alzheimer's Disease Research Center

State of California Alzheimer's Research and Clinical Center

Robert Joseph Bublitz
4400 Sevenoaks Court
Westlake Village, CA 91361

PARTICIPANT: Olive Mae Bublitz

Dear Mr. Bublitz,

Under the direction of Dr. Carol Miller, a postmortem examination of the brain has been completed on Olive Mae Bublitz. Enclosed please find a copy of the Neuropathology Summary Report of that examination.

The pathology report indicates that Mrs. Bublitz had a final primary diagnosis of definite Alzheimer's disease, which is consistent with her clinical diagnosis. She had secondary diagnoses of arteriolarsclerosis and atherosclerosis, which are thickening of arterial walls and plaques in the blood vessels that interfere with circulation.

We are most grateful for your generous contribution to medical science and participation in our vital research project concerning Alzheimer's disease and related illnesses here at the University of Southern California. If you have any questions, or if we can be of further assistance, please contact our office at (323) 442-7680.

Sincerely,

Bryan Spann, D.O., Ph.D.
Assistant Professor of Clinical Neurology
University of Southern California

1510 San Pablo Street
HCC 600
Los Angeles,
California 90033-5405
Tel: 323 442 7600
Fax: 323 442 7601
e-mail:
gsc@usc.edu
web page:
www.usc.edu/memory

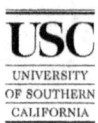

USC
UNIVERSITY
OF SOUTHERN
CALIFORNIA

Keck School of Medicine
University of Southern California

ADRC NEUROPATHOLOGY SUMMARY

Alzheimer's Disease Research Center

Department of Pathology

Carol A. Miller, M.D.
Director, Neuropathology Core
Professor of Pathology

Jenny K. Tang, M.S.
Program Specialist

Name of patient:	Bublitz, Olive	**Age:**	87
I.D.#:	8-3142-1	**Gender:**	F
Autopsy case #:	786	**Birthdate:**	08/08/1920
Pathologist:	Oblad, M.D.	**Time of death:**	22:45
Race:	Caucasian	**Time autopsy started:**	3:00
Date of death:	8/15/07	**Post-mortem interval:** 4 hrs/15 min.	
Date of autopsy:	8/16/07		

Clinical status: Premortem diagnosis: AD possible

Brain weight: 1000 gms. **Eyes taken?:** No

External Body: Normal

Skull: Normal

Dura: The dura is normal. There are no hemorrhages, nodules, discoloration or defects. The dural sinus is normal.

External Examination: The leptomeninges are thin and transparent. There is no congestion of the blood vessels, exudate hemorrhages, atrophy, swelling or softening of the brain. There is no herniation of the hippocampal uncus, cingulate gyrus or cerebellar tonsils.

Atrophy: __0_Frontal __1_Hippocampus _1_Temporal _1_Parietal _1_Occipital
(0 = None   1 = Mild   3 = Moderate   5 = Severe   9 = Not applicable)

Basilar vessels: There is a normal Circle of Willis and associated vessels with 75% atherosclerosis and no significant narrowing. There are no aneurysms, or AV malformations.

Coronal Sections: (Cerebrum, cerebellum, brainstem): In the cerebrum there is no swelling, atrophy, discoloration, hemorrhage, infarcts, lacunes, tumor or abscess. The cerebral ventricles are normal.

The basal ganglia and hypothalamus are normal. The cerebral white matter shows no periventricular or no diffuse pallor. The cerebellum is normal. The brainstem (midbrain, pons, medulla) are normal. There is no pallor of the substantia nigra, and no pallor of the locus ceruleus. The aqueduct Sylvius and IVth ventricle are normal.

Spinal Cord: Not taken **Stock?:** Yes

General Autopsy: CNS only

Gross Diagnosis: Mild cerebral atrophy

2011 Zonal Avenue
MCA 341A
Los Angeles,
California 90089
Tel: 323 442 1602
Fax: 323 442 1808

1

Appendix I: Olive's Autopsy Results

Name: Bublitz, Olive   **I.D. #** 8-3142-1   **Case #:** 786

0 = None   1 = Sparse (-5)   3 = Moderate (6-20)   5 = Frequent (21-30 or above)   9 = Not applicable

SILVER (Gallyas)

	Hippo. CA-1		Entorhinal cortex		Mid. Frontal	Sup./Mid. Temporal	Inferior parietal	Primary visual	Visual Assoc.
	LGB	UNCUS	LGB	UNCUS					
1. Neuritic plaques with or without cores	5	5	3	3	1	5	3	5	5
2. Neurofibrillary tangles	3	5	5	5	1	1	1	0	0
3. Neuropil threads	3	3	3	1	1	1	1	1	1

THIOFLAVIN

	Hippo. CA-1		Entorhinal cortex		Mid. Frontal	Sup./Mid. Temporal	Inferior parietal	Primary visual	Visual assoc.
	LGB	UNCUS	LGB	UNCUS					
1. Diffuse plaques	3	5	3	3	5	5	5	3	3
2. Immature (neuritic, no core)	3	3	5	5	3	3	3	3	5
3. Mature (neuritic, with core)	1	3	3	3	3	3	3	5	5
4. Neurofibrillary tangles	3	5	5	5	1	1	1	1	1

5. Vascular Amyloid	Area 22	Area 17
Parenchymal	0	0
Meningeal	0	0

None

Grade I	Amyloid restricted to a rim around normal/atrophic smooth muscle cells
Grade II	Media replaced by amyloid and thicker than normal, but no evidence of blood leakage
Grade III	Extensive amyloid deposition with focal vessel wall fragmentation and at least one focus of PV leakage (hemosiderin/hematoidin)
Grade IV	Extensive amyloid deposition and fibrinoid necrosis, micro aneurysms, mural thrombi, lumen with lumen or inflammation.

2

Name: Bublitz, Olive   I.D. #:   8-3142-1   Case #:   786

ANTI-SYNUCLEIN

	Midbrain	Hippocampus CA-1	Entorhinal cortex		Mid. Frontal	Sup./Mid. Temporal	Primary visual
7. Lewy bodies	9	9	9	9	9	9	9

MICROSCOPE (H & E)

	Hippocampus CA-1		Entorhinal cortex		Mid. frontal	Sup./Mid. Temporal	Inferior Parietal	Primary visual	Visual assoc.
	LGB	UNCUS							
Granulovacuolar degeneration	3	3							
Hirano bodies	1	1							
Neuronal loss	1	1	0	0	0	0	0	0	0
Gliosis	1	3	3	3	3	1	3	3	3
Pick bodies	0	0	0	0	0	0	0	0	0
Lewy bodies	0	0	0	0	0	0	0	0	0
Balloon cells	0	0	0	0	0	0	0	0	0

SUBSTANTIA NIGRA

Lewy bodies	0
Neuronal loss	0
Gliosis	0
Pigmentary incontinence	1

VASCULAR CHANGES

Arteriosclerosis in cerebral vessels?   Yes

Arteriolarsclerosis in cerebral vessels?   Yes

Other microscopic vascular disease?   No

Microinfarcts which are seen grossly?   No

White matter pallor with oligodendroglial loss?
    Anterior deep white matter?
    Posterior deep white matter?   Yes, posterior white matter pallor, focal

3

Appendix I: Olive's Autopsy Results

Name: Bublitz, Olive   **I.D. #** 8-3142-1   **Case #:** 786

1. **Microscopic exam:** H & E stained sections show moderate gliosis in the neocortex. Focal, mild, white matter pallor was seen in the anterior and posterior deep white matter. There is neuronal granulovacuolar degeneration in the CA1 region of the hippocampus. The midbrain shows mild pigmentary incontinence in the substantia nigra, without Lewy body changes. Gallyas and thioflavin S stains reveal frequent neuritic plaques and rare neurofibrillary tangles in the neocortex, frequent neuritic plaques and frequent neurofibrillary tangles in the CA1 region of the hippocampus. There are no amyloid protein deposits in meningeal or parenchymal blood vessels. The clinical history of dementia (CDR=3), and neuropathological changes are consistent with a diagnosis of definite Alzheimer's disease according to modified CERAD criteria. Using Reagan/NIA criteria, there is a high likelihood of a diagnosis of AD. Other pathological changes include focal microscopic extravascular old hemorrhage, moderate atherosclerosis of basilar artery, and moderate arteriolosclerosis of the cerebrum.

2. **Final diagnosis:**   (Primary Dx.)   Alzheimer's disease, definite
                                                (Braak & Braak score = V)

                             (Secondary Dx.)   Basilar vessels, atherosclerosis, severe
                                                Arteriolosclerosis of cerebrum, moderate

Carol A. Miller, M.D.
Carol A. Miller, M.D.
Chief Pathologist, ADRC
Director, ADRC Neuropath. Core

1-10-08
Date of Signature

4

Appendix J: Collage of Olive's Life

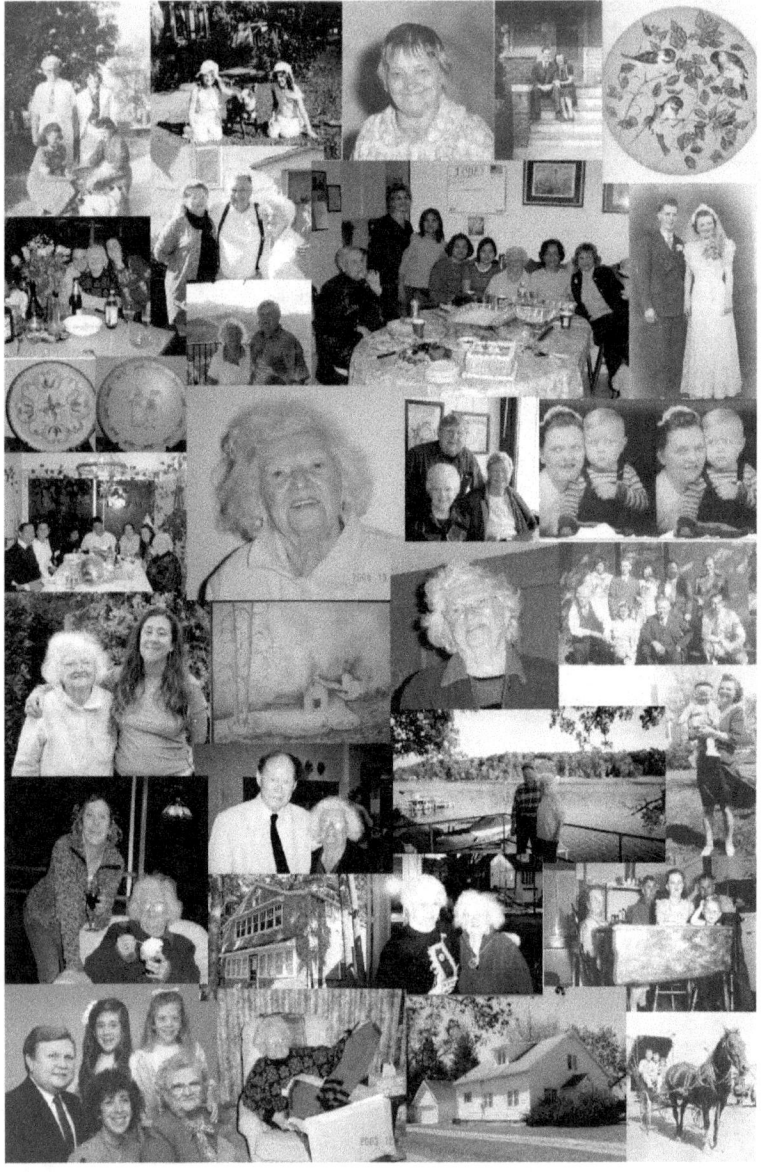

Appendix K: Olive's Obituary

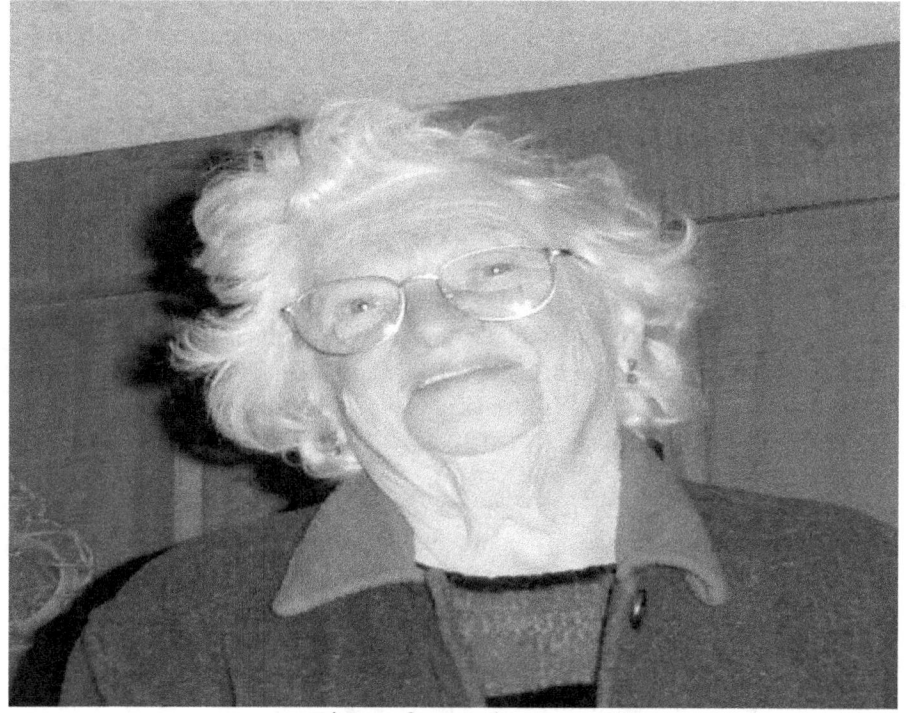

Picture from February 1, 2004

August 5, 1920 to August 15, 2007

Olive Mae Bublitz, age 87, who lived most of her life in Elkhorn, WI died at 10:45 p.m. Wednesday, August 15, 2007, at Leisure Living, Agoura Hills, CA after a long struggle against the indignities of Alzheimer's Disease. Olive was born August 5, 1920, in Burlington, Wisconsin to Joe and Evelyn Skotzke. She was raised and educated in Shorewood, a northern suburb of Milwaukee, Wisconsin. Olive met her husband, Bob, while she was visiting her relatives, the Steiners, who lived down the block from Grandma Tina Bublitz on Page Street. Olive and Bob Bublitz were married April 19, 1941, in Elkhorn, Wisconsin. Olive and Bob enjoyed a happy productive marriage for thirty-two years until Bob's sudden fatal heart attack November, 1973.

Alzheimer's--What My Mother's Caregiving Taught Me

The focal points of Olive's life were her family, friends, hobbies, and home. Olive worked in the musical instrument case manufacturing business founded by her brother-in law, Bill, and later owned by Olive and her husband, Bob, before selling the business to G. LeBlanc Corporation during the late sixties. Olive and Bob built their own home with the help of relatives and friends at 217 West Page Street in the early 1940s. Olive was active in TOPS, American Legion Auxiliary, a 4H Leader, a member of the First Evangelical Lutheran Church, and the Millard Community Church. Olive was an accomplished artist, enjoyed walking, rose mauling, crafts, collecting and restoring antiques, genealogy, playing the organ, enjoying a good game of cards, organizing and participating in family reunions, cooking, fishing and spending time at her Lauderdale Lake Cottage. Few people have fried as many fish from Lauderdale Lake as Ollie. Olive did not start painting until after her husband Bob's death; however, she completed approximately fifty paintings between 1975 and 2000. Olive studied painting with local artists, Elma and Thelma Olsen, and Gateway Instructors. Olive worked primarily in oils from the photographs she took of local barns, wildlife and rural scenes. Olive will long be remembered for her culinary skills, genealogy work, her beautiful detailed oil paintings, her happy smile and friendly outgoing personality.

Olive is survived by her only child, Bob Bublitz, Westlake Village, California sister, Elizabeth (Betty) Campagna, Milwaukee, WI and two grandchildren, Aubrey Bublitz, Santa Cruz, CA and Shelby Bublitz, Sherman Oaks, CA. She is further survived by many nieces, nephews, other relatives, and friends. Olive was preceded in death by her loving husband Bob Bublitz and her parents.

Visitation will be held at the First Evangelical Lutheran Church, 415 Devendorf Street, Elkhorn, WI 53121, Phone: 262-723-4191 on Friday, September 7th from 12:00 to 2:00 followed by a church service at 2:00 and graveside service. A late afternoon luncheon will be served at the church following the graveside services. Burial will be alongside her husband at Roselawn Memory Gardens, 3045 State Road 67, Lake Geneva, WI 53147, Phone: 262-245-6959. A memorial service to Celebrate of Olive's Life will be held at her son's home in Westlake Village, CA, Sunday, November 11, 2007. Please rsvp for the memorial service.

Appendix L: Olive's Eulogy

I would like to share a couple of light incidences before I begin the Eulogy for my mother.

Olive's comment to caregiver in the presence of Granddaughter, Aubrey, January 2005:
On a trip Aubrey and I made to Leisure Living to visit mother, Caregiver Rose said, "Olive, don't you think you should have Aubrey bring her boyfriend by so you can check him out?" Olive, thought for a second, then said, "I am sure any man Aubrey introduces me to I will like."

Shelby's Fondest Memory of her Grandmother, Spring 2003:
Grandma Olive's youngest granddaughter, Shelby said her fondest memory was coming over to the house one night and picking up grandma to go out for dinner. When Olive got in Shelby's car, she turned to Shelby and said, "I don't want to go out for dinner, let's go get some ice cream." Shelby said ok and they enjoyed ice cream for dinner. Shelby said, "Now, in looking back, I think this is why I like ice cream so much."

On a more serious side:
What do you say about someone who gives your life meaning? What do you say about someone who is always there with support and understanding; someone who makes sacrifices so that your life will be better and more successful? This special person was my mother, Olive Mae Bublitz!

God blessed Mother and me by giving us five years and eight months of Olive's final days to say goodbye. I never had this opportunity with my father. The love from my parents and the fellowship from the Bublitz and Albright families served as the foundation for my life and accomplishments. It has been the most meaningful of all experiences for me!

It has been a long, agonizing sixty-eight months watching my mother go from stubbornly insisting she could continue to live an independent life on her own, to needing more and more care as a result of Alzheimer's Disease and a series of strokes that took her mind and body. As Olive's only child, during this time, I felt like I was on a forced march, trying to do my best, but always feeling inadequate for the caregiving task.

Alzheimer's--What My Mother's Caregiving Taught Me

For many years mother traveled at Christmas time to our home, to enjoy holidays with us in Los Angeles and Portland, Oregon. In 1994 Mother made her last trip to our home in California. Other than her cardiology problems resulting from Rheumatic Fever, Mother always seemed healthy. She maintained a weight of 110 for thirty years, walked six miles each day and kept active with oil painting, genealogy, TOPS (Weight Loss Program), the Women's Legion Auxiliary, church activities, friends and relatives.

In July 1998 Olive fell at the Fireside Restaurant in Fort Atkinson where she, June Voss and Loraine Count had gone to eat before going to see a play. As mother was walking from the restaurant to the theater, she tripped, fell and suffered a concussion. Then, Thanksgiving weekend 2001, when Ollie had almost recovered from the concussion, she was involved in an auto accident near the old sheriff's office. A local doctor said that Mother had failed a mental test and recommended an MRI to see if there was brain damage from the latest accident. In January 2002 we went to The Mayo Clinic for Mother's routine cardiac check-up. The test showed stabilization of her cardiac problems and her cardiologists wished Ollie well. Next mother had an MRI and a half-day of full neuropsychological testing. During the consultation with a Neurologist, he indicated, the good news is there was no brain damage from the auto accident. However, the bad news is Olive had a fairly advanced case of osteoporosis, degenerative joint disease and Alzheimer's and would no longer be able to live by herself. In February 2002, after encouragement from Don and June Voss, Howard and Betty Dailey and my close friends, Kirt and Dixie Fiegle, Mother came to California to live with me.

Initially, Olive continued her daily walking and joined the Senior Concerns in Thousand Oaks, CA, a day care facility for dementia clients. Senior Concerns is a wonderful place with a full day of activities. Mother enjoyed her time at the Center. Friday night she enjoyed going to the Westlake Promenade and dancing with some of the Senior Concerns Caregivers.

As mother's condition declined, on November 12, 2004 she moved to Leisure Living in Agoura Hills. At Leisure Living mother received the best possible care available for an Alzheimer Patient. The facility is owned and managed by Ross and Pam Hashemi who are thoughtful and set high standards for care.

Appendix L: Olive's Eulogy

Before Olive moved to Leisure Living, Mother would stand in the bathroom doorway fifteen to twenty times a day and ask, "Where is the toilet?" When she was sleepy, she would ask, "Where should I lie down?" and conversations of any kind were difficult. Olive did not even remember that she had painted the beautiful landscapes and still lifes that hung proudly on the family room wall that she enjoyed viewing daily.

During the early part of the last five years, mother and I got to know each other once again and had many good times and conversations during her stay in California. During this time mother attended The Chinese New Year's Parade (February 2002), a Tony Bennett Concert at the Hollywood Bowl (August 2003) with the assistance of my good friend Jim Lindauer and a Willie Nelson concert (November 2003) with her granddaughters Aubrey and Shelby. During the early summer of 2004, Olive began to decline rapidly. Alzheimer's is known as the designer's disease because a patient's condition continually changes. A terrifying thing for a person to experience as they slowly but surely lose complete control of their mental faculties and associated physical capabilities. Alzheimer's is terrible disease to handle. One day a person's condition seems to improve. This gives you hope. The next day the condition worsens. Caregiving is very difficult, especially witnessing the constant decline of a loved one. First is the loss of short-term memory. Then follows decreased mobility as the disease affects the muscular system, increasing frailness. It is like watching the slow disappearance of a person. The physical and emotional demands are very difficult for loved ones and caregivers to handle. To make things worse, since the cause of death of an Alzheimer's patient is usually listed as pneumonia, heart attack, stroke, etc., it has the least amount of research, prevention and treatment options of any major cause of death. Only four medications are currently available for treatment and all are very ineffective. I urge everyone to support the national Alzheimer's Association in any way they are able to find a prevention or treatment for this dreadful disease.

Midway through this journey I was diagnosed with cancer at The Mayo Clinic and had surgery on Valentine's Day 2006 to remove the cells. A long recovery followed through April 2007. This made the journey even more difficult, but I have survived to be here today.

A couple of years ago, my mother sat in a sun lit room at Leisure Living and as I approached, she turned to a caregiver and said proudly, "This is my son,

Alzheimer's--What My Mother's Caregiving Taught Me

Bob." She reached for my hand and looked at me intently. She was fully aware that her only child was by her side. I said to her as I did many times, "Mother, you have been a good mother, a wife, sister, sister-in law, grandmother and a good person. You have many wonderful friends. You have enjoyed a full, happy life." I continued to tell her, "I love you" and thanked her for everything she did for me."

The woman who nearly died giving me birth, nurtured me from infancy to adulthood, taught me how to read, count, pray, cross Elkhorn Streets; whose belief in me provided the main motivation for major accomplishments in my life and protected me is no longer here. After being read the Lord's Prayer and the 23rd Psalm, Mother took a final deep breath and passed away gracefully and peacefully on Wednesday evening, August 15, 2007 at 10:45 pm PST at age 87.

With my mother's death, memories of the months of exhaustion, fear, self-doubt, second-guessing – and, yes, complaining, "When will this ever end?" instantly vanished. I have experienced the death of loved ones before (my dad, my grandmothers, aunts, uncles and friends), but never did it hurt like this. I am 65 years old and feel orphaned.

THESE HAVE BEEN THE MOST DIFFICULT, EMOTIONALLY DRAINING, PHYSICALLY AND FINANCIALLY CHALLENGING AND SPIRITUALLY DEMANDING AND IMPORTANT DAYS OF MY LIFE. I WANT TO EXPRESS OUR SINCERE GRATITUDE TO EVERYONE WHO HELPED US!

At this time, I want to personally thank everyone for attending mother's funeral and I want to thank the following individuals personally who during this difficult period provided me with support (please stand as I thank you):

- Don and June Voss for looking after mother's home and providing her with friendship, companionship, trust and emotional support through 2005.

- Pastor Grunewald, Nellie Kemp (deceased), and Darlene Schafer for their frequent visits with mother, which kept her spirits positive during the early phase in Elkhorn.

- Kirt Fiegel for helping us when things got very difficult; always listening and going out of his way to help.
- Steve and Chris Christianson, Rhonda Ford and Jeff Zimmerman, Elkhorn for being good neighbors who kept a watchful eye out for Olive and her property.
- Tom Knapp (deceased), who dependably cut the lawn and kept the sidewalks clear of snow.
- Granddaughters, Aubrey and Shelby, for their frequent visits and telephone conversations.
- California neighbors John Madison and Claire Belle Montenegro and friends Ken Bayus and Roger & Alice Eisele for their frequent visits and concern in California.
- Ross and Pam Hashemi & Staff, at Leisure Living, Agoura Hills; Maureen Symonds & Staff, Senior Concerns, Adult Day Center Director and staff; Betty Berry, Senior Concerns Advocate; Bonnie Olson & Staff, Buena Vista Hospice, General Manager; and Sue Lindeman, Moderator & Members; Thousand Oaks, CA Alzheimer's Support Group.
- Dr. Ed Portnoy, mother's initial attending physician, former neighbor and friend and Dr. Krumian, her final primary physician.

Finally, the most important thing that my mother and dad taught me during their life by their words and actions and that I want to share with you is, "Love is really everything!" and, "Love Will Give You Life!" My parents lived by this creed and enjoyed the love they shared and received in return from everyone.

Lastly, Mother, you have led a full, productive, joyous life. Many of us have enjoyed the beauty of your home, your fine culinary skills which increased our pleasure of being in your home, your oil paintings, your organ music and most of all, your friendship. Goodbye mother, you have left us with many precious memories. You will continue to live on in our hearts and minds from the many fond occasions we shared and enjoyed with you . . . Goodbye Mother, we love you dearly, may you rest in Peace.

Appendix M: Ken Bayus Condolence eMail

Dear Bob,

Thank you for sending this very thoughtful obituary to me. It was very nice to fill in the historical gaps I had in your mother's life.

I can honestly say that one of the best experiences, if not the best experience I've had since we renewed our friendship over 6 yrs ago, was meeting and getting to know your mom; what a delight she was. I remember meeting her for the very first time in your home; she was so friendly and kind to me. As I got to know her over the years, I realized what a special person she was.

Olive had a great sense of humor, which I prize greatly, and a very optimistic view on life. She was a fun person to be around and share stories with, and she had a loving and caring attitude towards all. I always enjoyed seeing all her paintings that you proudly displayed on your family room walls - it still amazes me how she was able to master the fine details and colors she displayed in her paintings. Olive also loved music and she loved to dance- I hope you didn't think I was too forward when, on many occasions, I twirled your mother around your living room. She made me very happy and I hope I gave her a little bit of joy too.

I thoroughly enjoyed the stories you and your mom told about growing up in Elkhorn, and how your mom had parties for all your friends. It was obvious to me she wanted everything to be just right for you. Bob I would have liked to have been at one of your parties, I know it would have been a blast.

I've also observed, along with you the terrible ravages of Alzheimer's in your mother's life and I have also observed your courageous fight to maintain her dignity and spirit. Even in her later years, Olive had a wonderful sparkle in her eyes that said volumes about her character and her life. She must have been quite a person in her younger days. You have been a wonderful son. I'm proud of you, and you should be proud of yourself.

Appendix M: Ken Bayus Condolence eMail

Bob, I know I mentioned to you on several occasions that my mother died when I was 4 yrs old, and frankly it wasn't until many, many years later, as an adult, that I realized what a huge void had been left in my life. Your relationship with your mom has made that even clearer to me. You've known your mother for 65 yrs, and I consider that a blessing; and now you will know her loving spirit for the rest of your life.

Bob, I extend my sincerest condolences to you and your family. May God bless you, and may he give comfort to you in your life.

Kindest regards,

Your friend,
Ken Bayus

Appendix N: Useful Alzheimer's References

Updated Resource List at:
http://www.www.alzheimerwhatmomscaretaughtme.com

Books

Mayo Clinic Guide to Alzheimer's Disease

Editor in Chief: Ronald Peterson M.D.
Hardcover: 350 pages
Publisher: Mayo Clinic Health Information, Rochester, MN;
Publication Date: January 28, 2006
Edition: 1st
ISBN-10: 1893005410
ISBN-13: 9781893005419

Book Description from Publisher

The Essential Resource for Treatment, Coping & caregiving. This book includes an explanation of the early signs an symptoms of dementia and how they differ from normal aging. The latest information is included on non-Alzheimer's forms of dementia, such as frontotemporal dementia, dementia with Lewy bodies and vascular cognitive impairment. Research advances in the understanding of mild cognitive impairment, a transitional stage between a transitional stage and dementia are described. Finally, included is an Action Guide for caregivers with tips and strategies for someone becoming a caregiver.

Mayo Clinic on Alzheimer's Disease

Editor in Chief: Ronald Peterson M.D.
Paperback: 192 pages
Publisher: Mayo Clinic Health Information, Rochester, MN;
Publication Date: September 1, 2002
Edition: 1st
ISBN-10: 1893005224
ISBN-13: 978-1893005228

Book Description from Publisher

Book covers how the brain functions and what can go wrong, conditions causing dementia, conditions that may accompany Alzheimer's, theories about causes, treatment of symptoms, tips for daily caregiving, care arrangements, and care costs.

Alzheimer's Early Stages: First Steps for Family, Friends and Caregivers

Author: Daniel Kuhn
Paperback: 304 pages
Publisher: Hunter House
Publication Date: March 27, 2003
Edition: 2nd
ISBN-10: 0897933974
ISBN-13: 978-0897933971

Book Description from Publisher

This edition includes the latest information on Alzheimer's risk factors, treatments, and prevention, as well as a new chapter, "Voices of Experience," composed of reflections by family members. It also provides information about new drugs approved since 1999 and the federal government's decision to cover counseling and other health-related services through Medicare.

Learning to Speak Alzheimer's: A Groundbreaking Approach for Everyone Dealing with the Disease

Author: Joanne Koenig Coste
Paperback: 256 pages
Publisher: Houghton Mifflin Harcourt
Publication Date: September 8, 2004
Edition Description: Reprint
ISBN-10: 1864710632
ISBN-13: 978-0618485178

Book Description From the Publisher

More than four million Americans suffer from Alzheimer's, and as many as twenty million have close relatives or friends with the disease. Revolutionizing the way we perceive and live with Alzheimer's, Joanne Koenig Coste offers a practical approach to the emotional well-being of both patients and caregivers that emphasizes relating to patients in their own reality. Her accessible and comprehensive method, which she calls habilitation, works to enhance communication between care partners and patients and has proven successful with thousands of people living with dementia. Learning to Speak Alzheimer's also offers hundreds of practical tips, including how to · cope with the diagnosis and adjust to the disease's progression · help the patient talk about the illness · face the issue of driving · make meals and bath times as pleasant as possible · adjust room design for the patient's comfort · deal with wandering, paranoia, and aggression.

Alzheimer's Action Plan

Authors: P. Murali Doraiswamy, Lisa P. Gwyther & Tina Adler
Paperback: 496 pages
Publisher: St. Martin's Press
Publication Date: April 28, 2009
Edition Description: 1st
ISBN: 0312538715
ISBN-13: 9780312538712

Book Description From the Publisher

This groundbreaking book combines the expertise of a world-class physician and an award-winning social worker to tell families everything they need to know about brain health and the early stages of memory loss, including how and why to intervene, the most (and least) effective treatments, practical strategies to optimize quality of life, and new research on prevention and care.

The Long Goodbye

Author: Patti Davis, President Ronald Reagan's daughter
Paperback: 224 pages
Publisher: Penguin Group (USA)
Publication Date: September 2005
Edition Description: Reprint
ISBN-10: 0452286875
ISBN-13: 978-0452286870

Book Description from Publisher

Patti Davis describes losing her father to Alzheimer's disease, saying goodbye in stages, helpless against the onslaught of a disease that steals what is most precious–a person's memory. "Alzheimer's," she writes, "snips away at the threads, a slow unraveling, a steady retreat; as a witness all you can do is watch, cry, and whisper a soft stream of goodbyes."

"Where's My Shoes?" My Father's Walk Through Alzheimer's

Author: Brenda Avadian
Paperback: 296 pages
Publisher: North Star Books

Publication Date: May 2005
Edition Description: 2nd
ISBN-10: 0963275240
ISBN-13: 978-0963275240

Book Description from Publisher

The heartfelt and uplifting story of a daughter's commitment to care for her father as the grip of Alzheimer's gradually controls his life. A poignant and sometimes humorous story that gives comfort to caregivers of dementia patients and the elderly.

Where's my Shoes? was written to increase the caregivers' strengths, insights and awareness of their options and to reduce the feelings of loneliness that can overwhelm the families involved. The book details specific suggestions for Alzheimer's caregivers and confronts issues and emotions all caregivers face

Alzheimer's, a Love Story: One Year in My Husband's Journey

Author: Ann Davidson
Hardcover: 224 pages
Publisher: Carol Publishing Corporation
Publication Date: June 1997
Edition Description: 1st
ISBN-10: 1559724188
ISBN-13: 978-1559724180

Book Description From the Publisher

In 1990, Ann Davidson's husband, Julian, a prominent physiology professor at Stanford Medical School, was diagnosed with Alzheimer's disease. He was fifty-nine. "I'm no longer intelligent", he told her later, "but, please let's enjoy our life together while I can still talk."

This is the gripping memoir of one critical year when Ann and her husband learned to live with his increasing dementia. It is the story of loyalty in the face of uncertainty and loss.

Following her husband's diagnosis, desperate for information, Ann felt terrified by what she read. Alzheimer's pamphlets were grim, mainly describing later stages in the long progression of the disease. The personal accounts she found usually did not explore emotions or create full pictures of daily life. And communication problems, so devastating in Alzheimer's, were glossed over.

Alzheimer's, A Love Story, offers fifty-six vignettes, each telling a complete story. The vignettes progress from Ann and Julian's initial confusion and anger, through adjustments with moments of humor and joy, to increasing acceptance and an odd sort of peace. They vow to go down this road with love and grace.

This stunning, touching book is full of visual detail and startlingly honest dialogue, providing comfort for people with a spouse, a relative, or a friend with Alzheimer's.

Final Gifts: Understanding the Special Awareness, Needs, and Communications of the Dying

Authors: Maggie Callanan & Patricia Kelley
Paperback: 231 pages
Publisher: Bantam Books
Publication Date: 1992
Edition Description: Reprint
ISBN-10: 0553378767
ISBN-13: 978-0553378764

Book Description from Publisher

Final Gifts has become a classic. In this moving and compassionate book, hospice nurses Maggie Callanan and Patricia Kelley share their intimate experiences with patients at the end of life, drawn from more than twenty years experience tending the terminally ill.

Through their stories we come to appreciate the near-miraculous ways in which the dying communicate their needs, reveal their feelings, and even choreograph their own final moments; we also discover the gifts—of wisdom, faith, and love—that the dying leave for the living to share.

Filled with practical advice on responding to the requests of the dying and helping them prepare emotionally and spiritually for death, Final Gifts shows how we can help the dying person live fully to the very end.

Awakening from Grief: Finding the Road Back to Joy

Author: John E. Welshons
Paperback: 232 pages
Publisher: New World Library; 2 Sub edition (August 1, 2003)
Publication Date: August 2003
Edition Description: 2nd
ISBN-10: 1930722184
ISBN-13: 978-1930722187

Book Description from Publisher

In this remarkable book, John Welshons weaves together his own personal awakening with those of others he's counseled to create a deeply felt and beautifully expressed primer on dealing with grief. Grieving, says Welshons, offers a unique opportunity to develop deeper and fuller life experiences, to embrace pain in order to open the heart to joy. Written for those who have experienced any kind of loss — death, divorce, or disappointment — this book offers reasonable, reassuring thinking on dealing with the death of loved ones and ourselves, finding the inner gifts that promote healing, and much more. Awakening from Grief takes a rare and compelling positive look at a subject needlessly viewed as one of the most negative in life. This is a persuasive primer on drawing the joy out of grief.

Walking: The Ultimate Exercise for Optimum Health

Authors: Andrew Weil & Mark Fenton
2 CD 's (2 hours, 15 minutes)
Publisher: Sounds True, Incorporated
Publication Date: January 2006
Edition Description: 1st
ISBN-10: 1591794099
ISBN-13: 978-1591794097

CD Description from Publisher

Most of us enjoy walking, but not everyone knows how to turn this simple exercise into one of the most powerful self-healing tools known to medicine. On Walking: The Ultimate Exercise for Optimum Health, Dr. Andrew Weil joins Mark Fenton, the nation's foremost expert on walking, for an invigorating 2-CD program that gives you all the tools needed to begin a daily walking practice. On Part One, Dr. Weil and Mark Fenton explain the proven ways in which walking helps you look and feel younger, reduce stress, improve immune function, achieve your ideal weight, and more. On Part Two, you get walking with a fully programmable workout that features two warm-up options and five intensifying sessions, paced by cadence cues and motivating tips for each phase. There are dozens of resources on walking for better health but none with the ultimate walking coach alongside America's most trusted complementary health-care physician. Whether you're a seasoned walking enthusiast looking for an edge or taking your first steps toward a healthier tomorrow, with Walking, anyone can put their best foot forward to make the most of this enjoyable and life-changing exercise.

Dr. Andrew Weil's Mind-Body Tool Kit
Publisher: Sounds True Inc.
Kit Contents: 2 CD 's (2 hours, 15 minutes) 1 Workbook (52 pages) 25 Card 's
Date Published: January 01, 2006
ISBN-10: 1-59179-410-2
ISBN-13: 978-1-59179-410-3

Product Description from Publisher
Experience Self-Healing with Proven Techniques-Breathwork, Meditation, Guided Imagery & Sound Therapy

Discover Your Own Self-Healing Powers with Mind-Body Tools from Dr. Andrew Weil. The evidence is overwhelming: you can tap the power of your mind to directly influence your health, using clinically proven tools that anyone can master. With Dr. Andrew Weil's Mind-Body Tool Kit, listeners join the best-selling author of Spontaneous Healing (Ballantine, 1996) along with three renowned colleagues and friends—all leading specialists in alternative medicine—to experience a potent prescription of self-healing practices. This information-packed "integrative medicine chest" includes an in-depth 52-page interactive workbook and 25 Mind-Training Cards designed to support a daily practice. Step by step, users will learn an empowering four-part series of mind-body techniques: • Breathing—Dr. Weil reveals "the master key to self healing" • Meditation—Dr. Jon Kabat-Zinn introduces listeners to the oldest and most effective system for calming the mind • Guided Imagery—Dr. Martin Rossman invites us to heal the body with this effective and easy-to-learn skill • Sound Therapy—Pioneering music therapist Kimba Arem leads a complete sound-healing journey to rejuvenate and balance our physiology and mind states "Your mind can elicit a healing response when even conventional medicine has proven ineffective," explains Dr. Weil. Here are the self-healing mind-body tools to start optimizing your health today— and for the rest of your life—with Dr. Andrew Weil's Mind-Body Tool Kit. Note: Includes material from Breathing, Meditation for Optimum Health, Self-Healing with Guided Imagery, and Self-Healing with Sound and Music.

Videos

On Our Own Terms: Bill Moyer on Dying
Run Time: Six hours
Original Release Date: 2000
Studio: Films for Humanities and Science

Studio VHS Description
The following is a very useful internet site:
http://www.pbs.org/wnet/onourownterms/about/index.html

From the back of the box "On Our Own Terms" presents remarkable human stories of the dying and their wishes to meet life's ultimate passage with compassion, comfort, and dignity. Emmy award winning journalist Bill Moyers looks at how we die in America, providing an intimate window into the daily experience of patients, their families, and their caregivers, including the decisions they face and the changes they undergo. Along with this deeply personal perspective, we meet the medical, legal, and public policy experts who offer suggestions for improving conditions for terminal patients. This item is a box set of four individual videos, including:
Program One: Living With Dying
Program Two: A Different Kind of Care
Program Three: A Death of One's Own
Program Four: A Time to Change

The Notebook
Director: Nick Cassavetes, Actors: James Garner, Gena Rowlands, Rachel McAdams, Ryan Gosling, Anthony-Michael Q. Thomas Starring: James Garner, Gena Rowlands
DVD Release Date: February 8, 2005
Run Time: 123 minutes
Studio: New Line Home Video

Studio DVD Description
The Notebook is an epic love story centered around an older man who reads aloud to an older, invalid woman whom he regularly visits. From a faded

notebook, the old man's words bring to life the story about a couple who is separated by World War II, and is then passionately reunited, seven years later, after they have taken different paths. Though her memory has faded, his words give her the chance to relive her turbulent youth and the unforgettable love they shared.

As teenagers, Allie (Rachel McAdams) and Noah (Ryan Gosling) begin a whirlwind courtship that soon blossoms into tender intimacy. The young couple is quickly separated by Allie's upper-class parents who insist that Noah isn't right for her. Several years pass, and, when they meet again, their passion is rekindled, forcing Allie to choose between her soul mate and class order. This beautiful tale has a particularly special meaning to an older gentleman (James Garner) who regularly reads the timeless love story to his aging companion (Gena Rowlands).

Pictures of Hollis Woods
Actors: Sissy Spacek, Alfre Woodard, Jodelle Ferland
Run Time: 98 minutes
Original Release Date: 2007
Source: Hallmark Hall of Fame

Studio DVD Description
Having run away from a succession of foster homes, a 12-year-old girl resorts to desperate measures to stay with the eccentric retired teacher who's made her feel like she's finally in the place where she belongs.

Iris
Director: Richard Eyre Cast: Judi Dench, Kate Winslet, Hugh Bonneville, Jim Broadbent
Original Release: 2001
Source: MIRAMAX

Studio DVD Description
Here's the powerful true story based on John Bayley's novels that earned Jim Broadbent an Academy Award(R) for Best Supporting Actor and Academy Award(R) nominations for Best Actress Judi Dench and Best Supporting Actress Kate Winslet (IRIS, 2001). Judi Dench (SHAKESPEARE IN LOVE) and Kate Winslet (TITANIC) bring to the screen one of the most extraordinary women of the 20th century, celebrated English author Iris Murdoch. As told by her unlikely soulmate, husband John Bayley, Iris first became known as a brilliant young scholar at Oxford whose boundless spirit dazzled those around her. Then, during her remarkable career as a novelist

and philosopher, she continued to prove herself a woman ahead of her time. Even in later life, as age and illness robbed Iris of her remarkable gifts, nothing could diminish her immense influence or weaken the bond with her devoted husband.

Away from Her
Director: Sarah Polley Cast: Julie Christie, Gordon Pinsent, Olympia Dukakis, Michael Murphy & Wendy Crewson
Run Time: 110 minutes
Original Release Date: 2006
Source: LIONS GATE

Studio DVD Description
Married for almost 50 years, Grant's (Gordon Pinsent) and Fiona's (Julie Christie) commitment to each other appears unwavering. Their daily life is filled with tenderness and humor; yet this serenity is broken by Fiona's increasingly evident memory loss - and her restrained references to a past betrayal. For a while, the couple is able to casually dismiss these unwelcome changes. But when neither Fiona nor her husband can deny any longer that she is being consumed by Alzheimer's disease, the couple is forced to wrenchingly redefine the limits of their love and loyalty - and face the complex, inevitable transition from lovers to strangers.

Alzheimer's Disease Internet Sites

ORGANIZATION NAME & GENERAL INFORMATION (IN ALPHABETICAL ORDER)	URL AND CONTACT INFORMATION
Alzheimer's Society is a United Kingdom care and research charity for people with dementia and their caregivers. It is a membership organization, which works to improve the quality of life of people affected by dementia in England, Wales and Northern Ireland.	http://www.alzheimers.org.uk
Alzheimer's & Dementia: The Journal of the Alzheimer's Association	http://www.alzheimersanddementia.org
Alzheimer's Association National Office is a non-profit American voluntary health organization which	www.alz.org 225 N. Michigan Ave., Floor 17 Chicago, IL 60601

ORGANIZATION NAME & GENERAL INFORMATION (IN ALPHABETICAL ORDER)	URL AND CONTACT INFORMATION
focuses on care, support and research for Alzheimer's disease.	
Alzheimer's Disease Education Referral Center (ADEAR) Center. Site will help you find current, comprehensive Alzheimer's disease (AD) information and resources from the National Institute on Aging (NIA).	www.nia.nih.gov/Alzheimers/ National Institute on Aging U.S. National Institutes of Health Building 31, Room 5C27 31 Center Drive, MSC 2292 Bethesda, MD 20892 Phone: 301-496-1752
Alzheimer's Disease International (ADI) is the umbrella organization of Alzheimer Associations around the world. ADI aim is to help establish and strengthen Alzheimer associations throughout the world, and to raise global awareness about Alzheimer's disease and all other causes of dementia.	http://www.alz.co.uk/
Alzheimer's Foundation of America	http://www.alzfdn.org 322 8th Ave., 7th Fl. New York, NY 10001
Alzheimer's Research Trust Leading UK Research Charity for Dementia	http://www.alzheimersresearch. org.uk/ The Stables, Station Road, Great Shelford Cambridge, CB22 5LR, UK
AlzOnline; Caregiver Support Online, Center for Telehealth and Healthcare Communications at the University of Florida.	http://alzonline.phhp.ufl.edu/
American Heart Association	http://www.americanheart.org American Heart Association National Center 7272 Greenville Avenue Dallas, TX 75231

Appendix N: Useful Alzheimer's References

ORGANIZATION NAME & GENERAL INFORMATION (IN ALPHABETICAL ORDER)	URL AND CONTACT INFORMATION
	1-800-242-8721
Family Caregiver Alliance Family Caregiver Alliance (FCA) seeks to improve the quality of life for caregivers through education, services, research and advocacy.	http://www.caregiver.org National Center on Caregiving 180 Montgomery Street Suite 1100 San Francisco, CA 94104 (415) 434-3388 (800) 445-8106
HealthGrades (NASDAQ: HGRD), provides objective ratings of hospitals, nursing homes and home health agencies in the United States. The Company also provides detailed information on physicians, including name, address, phone number, years in practice, information on whether they are board certified, whether they are free of state and federal sanctions and many other items.	http://www.healthgrades.com
Mayo Clinic	http://www.mayoclinic.com/ Mayo Clinic (Main Site) 200 First St. S.W. Rochester, MN 55905 General Telephone Number: (507) 284-2511 Arizona - Scottsdale / Phoenix Branch 13400 East Shea Blvd. Scottsdale, AZ 85259 (480) 301-8000 Florida - Jacksonville Branch San Pablo Road Jacksonville, FL 32224 (904) 953-2000

ORGANIZATION NAME & GENERAL INFORMATION (IN ALPHABETICAL ORDER)	URL AND CONTACT INFORMATION
Medicaid Plans by State	http://www.medicaid-plans.com/medicaidplans7
MedlinePlus Health, authoritative information from the National Library of Medicine (NLM), the National Institutes of Health (NIH), and other government agencies and health-related organizations.	http://medlineplus.gov/
National Center for Disease Control and Prevention	http://www.cdc.gov/
National Academy of Elder Law Attorneys, Inc.	http://www.naela.com/
National Cell Repository for Alzheimer's Disease	http://ncrad.iu.edu/ 1-800-526-2839 email at alzstudy@iupui.edu.
National Human Genome Research Institute (NHGRI)	http://www.genome.gov
National Institute of Neurological Disorders and Stroke	http://www.ninds.nih.gov National Institutes of Health Bethesda, MD 20892
Neurobiology of Aging Journal	http://www.neurobiologyofaging.org/issues
Quicken® Home Inventory Manager, Quicken® Personal Financial Manager, To inventory assets and personal property	http://quicken.intuit.com/ http://quicken.intuit.com/personal-finance/home-inventory.jsp
Quicken® WillMaker	http://nolo.com or http://quicken.intuit.com/
Science Daily	http://www.sciencedaily.com/videos/2006/0303-predicting_alzheimers.htm
The Journal of Alzheimer's Disease (often abbreviated JAD) is an international multidisciplinary journal published by IOS Press covering the	http://www.j-alz.com/

Appendix N: Useful Alzheimer's References

ORGANIZATION NAME & GENERAL INFORMATION (IN ALPHABETICAL ORDER)	URL AND CONTACT INFORMATION
etiology, pathogenesis, epidemiology, genetics, behavior, treatment and psychology of Alzheimer's disease. The journal publishes research reports, reviews, short communications, hypotheses, book reviews, and letters-to-the-editor and is dedicated to providing an open forum for original research that will expedite our fundamental understanding of Alzheimer's disease.	
The National Alzheimer's Coordinating Center (NACC) was established by the National Institute on Aging in 1999 to facilitate collaborative research among the 29 NIA-funded Alzheimer's Disease Centers (ADCs) nationwide. NACC developed and maintains a large relational database of standardized clinical and neuropathological research data collected from each ADC, and this database provides a valuable resource for both exploratory and explanatory Alzheimer's disease research. The center is located on the campus of the University of Washington	http://www.alz.washington.edu/ 4311 11th Ave NE, #300 Seattle, WA 98105 phone: (206) 543-8637; fax: (206) 616-5927 email: naccmail@u.washington.edu
The National Institute on Aging (NIA) is a division of the U.S. National Institutes of Health (NIH), located in Bethesda, Maryland. The NIA leads a broad scientific effort to understand the nature of aging and to extend the healthy, active years of life. Designated by NIA as the primary Federal agency on Alzheimer's disease research.	http://www.nia.nih.gov/

About The Author

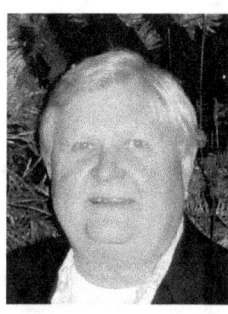

Robert Bublitz, Alzheimer's author and popular expert speaker gained extensive knowledge from his research on Alzheimer's disease and experience caring for his mother. Bob was working at his career in marketing and sales in electronics when Olive was diagnosed with Alzheimer's Disease. Being an only child, Bob dropped everything and accepted full responsibility for his mother's health care. Bob was determined to make his mother's final days as pleasant as possible.

This book is the result of the knowledge and experience which Bob shares with others to lighten the burden they face with this disease. Bob earned a Bachelor's degree from Northland College, a Master's degree from the University of Arizona and the equivalent of an electrical engineering degree from numerous classes during his thirty year career in integrated circuit design.

Bob is available for speaking engagements, workshops or consulting. Please see the book's internet site for more information:
http://www.www.alzheimerwhatmomscaretaughtme.com and

Index

Index